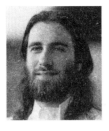Swami Purnachaitanya is an author, speaker, and spiritual guide to many around the world. He is a sought-after teacher of yoga, meditation and mantras, and an enthralling storyteller. Swamiji was born in the Netherlands to a Dutch father and an Indian mother, who played a central role in kindling in him a keen interest in the spiritual practices, cultures and philosophies of the East. The defining moment in his life came at the age of sixteen, when he met Gurudev Sri Sri Ravi Shankar, the founder of the Art of Living, in whom he recognized his spiritual Master.

After completing his university studies in Indology with a specialization in Sanskrit, he left the Netherlands and moved to The Art of Living International Centre in Bengaluru, India to master the Vedic knowledge, rituals and recitation of mantras and Vedic hymns. He received his title Swami (monk) as an acknowledgement of his high state of consciousness and commitment to dedicating his life to serving others. Purnachaitanya is the name given to him by his Master, meaning he whose consciousness (*chaitanya*) has fully blossomed (*purna*).

He is currently a Director of Programs for the Art of Living where he conducts a range of personal development trainings and oversees various service projects in India and Africa.

PRAISE FOR THE BOOK

'When the world around us is in turmoil, we need to look inward. Meditation is the tool that can give us the much-needed solace and inner strength.'
– Gurudev Sri Sri Ravi Shankar, world-renowned humanitarian, spiritual leader and peace ambassador

'Your emotional health has a direct impact on your physical health. *Looking Inward* allows you to identify the root cause of your stress, anxiety and other negative emotions and this book will enable you to address them with the help of meditation. Its beauty lies in its simplicity and clarity of thought. A must read for anyone looking to build meditation as a practise.' – Luke Coutinho, author and wellness guru

'In *Looking Inward*, Swami Purnachaitanya brings to the reader a beautiful handbook on meditation that one can safely practice and learn in their home. Given the state of the world we are in, everyone must read this book full of ancient wisdom presented in an easy-to-follow format.'
– Yash Birla, Indian industrialist Dated: 17th February 2022

Dear Swami Purnachaitanya,

My father had received a copy of your book Looking Inward, and was immersed in it when illness overtook him.

I know that, other than his Bible, his Book of Common Prayer, missal and hymn book, this was the only book that he took with him to the hospice where his life ended.

The prayer book, missal, hymnal and Bible are what he needed to be able to complete his daily cycle of prayers that we in the family knew as his office. The saying of the office was a routine in which he had engaged twice daily since he was ordained a priest in 1961. It was a habit that he continued throughout his life, and even severe illness had never prevented him from carrying it out.

He had prepared himself for death, and in many ways was looking forward to it, as he had turned more and more to the spiritual aspects of his being. I think that this book, that you gave him, made him accept the end with equanimity and complete nonchalance. He knew where he was going, and was ready to take the final steps. He was of good cheer, and I think that this book helped him to achieve that peace of mind, and ready his spirit / soul for its new adventure.

Thank you for having given him this great gift, and for having helped him in his last days.

Kind regards,

Trevor Tutu, son of Archbishop Desmond Tutu

LOOKING INWARD

How to Find Calm in a Chaotic World

SWAMI
PURNACHAITANYA

Lagom

First published by Penguin Random House India 2021
This edition published in the UK in 2022 by Lagom
An imprint of Bonnier Books UK
4th Floor, Victoria House, Bloomsbury Square,
London, WC1B 4DA

Owned by Bonnier Books
Sveavägen 56, Stockholm, Sweden

Hardback – 9781788706582
Ebook – 9781788706599

A CIP catalogue of this book is available from the British Library.

Designed by Envy Design Ltd

Printed and bound by Clays Ltd, Elcograf S.p.A

3 5 7 9 10 8 6 4 2

Every reasonable effort has been made to trace copyright holders of material
reproduced in this book, but if any have been inadvertently overlooked the
publishers would be glad to hear from them.

Some names, dates and places have been changed to protect the identity and
privacy of those who form part of the narrative.

Lagom is an imprint of Bonnier Books UK
www.bonnierbooks.co.uk

Contents

Introduction: A New Approach

The world as we know it is rapidly changing. Global warming, a pandemic, information spreading like wildfires, fake news, riots, and changing social structures and lifestyles. The magnitude and impact of these and so many other challenges we face affect our health, productivity, and finally, our happiness and inner peace. It is in times like these that most people could feel stressed, acutely anxious and in some cases, even depressed. And it is now more than ever that we need to look inward for strength, focus and peace of mind.

In this practical guide, I will help you on your personal journey towards finding the source of your anxiety, stress and restlessness, as well as guide you how to address and overcome them, using meditation to soothe distracted thoughts and refocus your energy to being present in the moment while also building resilience.

The idea is to acknowledge the changing outside world while strengthening your inner energy reserves to better cope with it. It does not involve you running away or pretending all the bad stuff never happened, nor does it involve you trying to feel better by just imagining everything is actually okay. It is about finally learning how our mind works, and how to manage it, so that you can transcend it and access the one source of peace, happiness and support that remains unaffected and unchanged.

For years I have been teaching meditation programs of The Art of Living to people from all backgrounds, ranging from indigenous people in the most interior parts of the North Eastern region in India, to top executives and CEOs of leading international corporates, from college students and homemakers to successful artists and politicians; and all have greatly benefitted from the practice in various aspects of their lives. Realizing the increasing need for this valuable knowledge to reach the many people looking for an effective way to deal with life and come out on top, I decided to write this book.

The book you are holding in your hands right now contains many of the most valuable insights and techniques that I have learned and realized over the last twenty years of my meditation practice under the guidance of my master, Gurudev Sri Sri Ravi Shankar, a true realized meditation master of our times. I am offering my learning and experience to anyone who is sincerely interested in finally looking a little closer at life and trying a new approach, or rather a very ancient one, to deal with many of life's challenges and how they affect our health, happiness and peace of mind. Sharing this knowledge with you in an easy-to-understand-and-apply language and methodology, I provide you with a practical approach to manage your mind, and finally master it.

There are many misconceptions and wrong notions when it comes to meditation nowadays, as in the last few decades it has found itself transitioning from what was, by many, perceived as a strange occult practice, that was associated with scarcely-clad yogis in the Himalayas, to the latest trend of mental fitness for the hip and successful, with an increasing number of mobile apps that promise you peace of mind in as little as three minute 'instant' meditations. On top of that, many embraced the term 'mindfulness' as the new and much more secular word for meditation, making it easier to market to both the masses and corporate honchos, not realizing that meditation and mindfulness are really not the same, and in some ways even exactly opposite to each other.

I felt it was high time, therefore, to write a book that clears many of these misconceptions and wrong notions. One that allows anyone with an interest to start exploring meditation in a proper manner, and without getting caught up in either too much incense, or too little substance.

Meditation is an ancient, time-tested and very effective art of managing our mind and transcending it. It has countless benefits, ranging from how it impacts your social and professional life, to your personal health, happiness and sense of freedom and fulfilment. Trying to strip it from its context and tradition will not only be an injustice to the very masters who have preserved this knowledge till today but would also deprive the practice of some of its most effective and essential aspects.

At the same time, our modern world and lifestyle requires us to make this ancient wisdom and techniques available in a way that they can be easily understood, related to, and practiced by anyone who wishes to explore the manifold benefits it offers. This book will be your personal guide to understanding this profound practice for a healthier, happier and well-adjusted life.

This book is structured in a way that each chapter will teach you some of most important principles, to progress on the journey, and impart you the knowledge and know-how that will finally come together in your personal meditation practice. Many of the principles that you will learn in these pages will also make you more effective, efficient, and empathic in your day-to-day activities and help you to deal more skilfully with this abstract thing called the mind and all its tantrums. It will make your life easier, more enjoyable, and more fulfilling, but it will require you to read, understand, and practice what has been shared.

You will learn that meditation does not require a lot of focus or concentration, rather the opposite, and that it can actually be a joyful journey full of eye-openers. It is a journey from effort to effortlessness, from activity to stillness, and from stress, anxiety and frustration to a state of peace and tranquillity. One thing that I would like to emphasize though, is that meditation is so much more than just a solution to some of these problems that many of us face. And practicing it simply to overcome these problems would mean you may drop the practice when your mind or life has settled down again. I would rather encourage you to aim higher and think bigger. Meditation will give you all those benefits, but these are more like the side effects. The real treasure you can find inside lies beyond, and is only revealed to those who are really ready to look inward.

Come then, whether you are totally new to meditation, or have been practicing regularly or irregularly for many years. I invite you to embark on this fascinating journey with an open mind. When you are able to do this, I guarantee that you will learn and realize many things that can help you understand and deepen your meditation practice and enrich your life. After all, in today's modern world, meditation is not a luxury, it is a necessity, and the sooner we realize this, the better.

A mind without agitation . . . is meditation
A mind in the present moment . . . is meditation
A mind, which becomes 'no mind' . . . is meditation
A mind that has no hesitation, no anticipation . . .
    is meditation
A mind that has come back home, to the source . . .
    is meditation

— Gurudev Sri Sri Ravi Shankar

1

Yes, the World Is Changing

I picked up my phone and scrolled through my WhatsApp conversations. Ah, there it is, the number of my friend from Delhi. The Covid-19 pandemic had me locked in an apartment in Johannesburg for almost two months now. After India closed her borders and airports overnight, I had managed to travel to South Africa from Ghana at the last minute, before both countries also closed their borders. A friend in Johannesburg had kindly agreed to provide me a place to stay for as long as I needed – something I was grateful for as many have not been so fortunate during this sudden global shut-down of not just travel, but most aspects of our lives itself.

'Hey Samir, how have you been? I was remembering you all. How is your family?'

'Swamiji, so nice to hear from you! Things are okay, we are managing.' The tone of his voice sounded a little less

confident than the words he chose. 'My brother came back home, due to the lockdown. So, we are all together again.'

I have known Samir for quite a few years now, and we had become good friends. He is a professional photographer, who mostly shoots weddings – a huge industry in India, with plenty of opportunities if you are good at what you do. Samir got married a few years back, and his brother was going to be a father soon. Samir and his wife are living with his parents, and his brother temporarily moved to West Bengal some time ago for a good job opportunity there. They had all been saving money to get a bigger place as their apartment is small, especially now that both brothers were married. They bought a small plot of land in another part of Delhi and were planning to build a house there for the whole family. One floor would be for their parents to live, and one floor would be for Samir and his wife, with his brother occupying the last floor. This way, they would all have enough space to live comfortably. There had been some delays, as business had been slow, but the upcoming wedding season would have brought in sufficient money to finally start the work. They had all been dreaming of finally having their own place.

'How about the house? I forgot to ask you about that the last time we spoke. I remember you were planning to start the construction work any time now, right? But I guess it is delayed now with the lockdown?'

'Actually, Swamiji, it looks like we won't be able to start the construction. Not any time soon at least. We just got the news that my brother is losing his job, as the company is not *able to retain everyone in the current scenario, so we will need the money we had saved to manage our expenses. I have also not been able to earn anything the last few months as a photographer, and we do not know how much longer the lockdown will continue. Even when it opens up, it will take a lot of time before there will be any events like weddings again. Then too, people will have much less money to spend – it is a difficult time for everyone right now.' I paused for a moment, thinking of what to tell him. I pictured all of them living together in the small apartment – a place I knew personally as I had also stayed with them once in the past, when visiting Delhi. Considering that his sister-in-law was expecting a baby, it would become even more crowded and challenging.*

This is life. This is our life. We, more than often, don't realize it, but everything that we take for granted, or that we rely on, can change at any time. And this is nothing new of course; it has always been like that since time immemorial. Despite our sincerest efforts, life doesn't always go as planned, and it never ceases to surprise, be it for the better, or worse.

However, recent years have seen things change faster, and more radically, than many of us, and even our previous generation, would have known. I cannot speak for those who lived through the Second World War, but we are currently seeing a scenario that is affecting many people in almost similar ways, if not worse. It's no wonder that even eminent personalities and experts have not shied away from describing the Covid-19 pandemic as the 'Third World War' when explaining the impact it has had on people's lives. The United Nations (UN) has officially stated that the pandemic is the most challenging crisis the world has faced since the Second World War, and it is the worst crisis the UN has ever faced since her inception. 'It is not just a health crisis, it is a human crisis,' the UN chief António Guterres has warned, explaining that the economic impact will bring a recession that has been unparalleled in recent times. The UN's food relief agency has warned of a possible 265 million people being pushed to the brink of starvation, fearing a global famine of biblical proportions. The UN has also projected that around 200 million people may lose their jobs due to the pandemic, contributing to a total number of about 800 million people across the world being pushed below the poverty line, not being able to meet their basic needs. An Oxfam report published before the G20 group of leading developed and developing nations, the International Monetary Fund and the World Bank, even said that by the time the pandemic is over, half of the world's population of 7.8 billion people could be living in poverty.

And to make matters worse, the pandemic is just one of the most recent developments that has shaken up the lives of people in countries across the world, leaving many desperately reaching for anything that could possibly stop them from falling – falling into despair, depression, or disillusion with life itself.

In the year that culminated in the announcement of this new virus that started spreading in China, we saw massive wildfires raging across Australia, as well as sudden violent protests in Hong Kong, the Middle East, and in various countries across South and Central America. A trade war between the United States and China had people worried all over the world, and climate change continues to have more catastrophic effects on our ecology. Natural calamities have hardly left any continent untouched, spanning from earthquakes and floods to cyclones and droughts. A recent example is the cyclone Amphan in East India that left thousands of people without roofs over their heads, and many tens of thousands more with damaged homes or crops, having destroyed large parts of coastal West Bengal, including Kolkata, in India, as well as parts of Bangladesh. It was claimed to be the most destructive cyclone to have hit the metropolitan and the entire region in the last 500 years and is said to have directly affected 70 per cent of the entire population of West Bengal.

Friends of mine in Argentina and Zimbabwe have seen their savings wither away as local economies started collapsing, leaving them without many options but to pray for better times, and they were not the only ones. We have seen economies stumbling across the world, sometimes falling as far as to border collapse, even in regions like Western Europe, some that are counted amongst the most developed countries in the world.

For me, it was surreal to see that even in our modern, developed and advanced societies, things could change overnight. To see our so-called civilized societies turn to violent protests, looting and experience a sudden economic collapse, reinforced something that the ancient scriptures of the East that I have studied have always warned us about: don't look for support in the ever-changing, as the nature of the world is change. The only true support and security can be found in the non-changing. And for that you need to look inward.

So, what is it that we look for to feel secure, that we look for to feel safe? Having a comfortable home? A good bank balance or pension? Good health, a large circle of friends? Social status, or recognition? Often, we only realize the importance of these things, when they suddenly fall away, and with it, our peace of mind, our sense of security, our happiness, and sometimes even our hope, or faith. And we are not really to blame, because this is how we were raised; this is what we were taught since childhood. We learnt that we should work hard so that we could get a good job, a nice house, a good circle of friends, and maybe even earn social status. We should also exercise and watch our diet a little so that we are healthy and strong. We were told that we should have all these, as they will provide us with the happy and secure life that we all aspire to. Because in the end we all want the same: to be happy, to be peaceful, to feel safe and secure, and to be free. It is what every commercial promises you, whether it is trying to sell you a new watch, a new car model, a certain shampoo, or a life insurance. This is why many are ready to sacrifice almost anything to attain that magical life where they don't have to worry about anything and they can live the life they dreamed of, because they can afford it. But then again, when you look a little closer, you will see that the people who are supposed to 'have it all' have almost all the same problems. They are also stressed, worried, insecure or anxious at times, and sometimes even more so than others!

Much too often, I open a newspaper to come across stories of people, even students, who have committed suicide over setbacks like a bad break-up or having failed an exam. Farmers committing suicide because they were not able to cope with the challenges and debts they were facing are sadly just one more example of this phenomenon. Depression numbers have continued to rise globally, which makes us wonder if our technological advancements and economic progress and development are taking us in the right direction.

No doubt, having a tidy sum in the bank or a good pension can help you take care of your needs, and maybe even leave you with enough to meet some of your wants. Good health, a nice group of friends to hang out with, and a steady job, all help us to feel happy, secure and free. But what if these suddenly fall away? Because as unlikely as it may have seemed earlier, it is now a reality for many across the world. How does one deal with that? How to remain unshaken, how to face such challenges? History has left us with stories of great people who faced adversities or opposition that may have seemed insurmountable, and yet they were able to keep moving ahead until, eventually, even emerging successful. How were they able to do that when they may have even lacked all these things that we may turn to for our support, or security? What gave them this strength?

A story comes to mind here that has stayed with me ever since I heard it many years ago. It relates an incident that is said to have taken place in the life of Alexander the Great, during his conquest of the known world. It is said that his teacher, Aristotle, had asked him, before he left Greece, to bring back a yogi from India, as they were known for their profound wisdom and esoteric teachings, even in those days. Having crossed the Himalayas and having reached India, Alexander heard about a great yogi who was rumoured to be living in the forest nearby.

Alexander sent one of his generals to go fetch the holy man and bring him to him. As the general approached the place where the yogi had supposedly taken up residence, he saw a man sitting in meditation, seemingly unaware of his surroundings. Approaching the yogi, the general made his presence known, but it was only after addressing him a few times that the yogi finally opened his eyes and spoke. The general told him to come with him, as the great Emperor Alexander the Great had summoned him. The yogi made it clear that he was not bothered, and he made it known to the general that he was disturbing his meditation and asked him to please leave him alone. The general was shocked with this answer. He tried persuading the yogi with many fine and precious gifts if he would accompany him to no avail. The general even threatened the yogi with dire consequences for his refusal to obey the Great Alexander's summons, but the latter had made up his mind, closed his eyes again, and did not move an inch.

Perplexed with this whole episode, the general returned to Alexander, and recounted his experience with the holy man. Furious but also intrigued that someone had so blatantly ignored his order, even when threatened, Alexander decided to go and see this yogi himself. Having come there, he told the yogi who he was, and that he better obey him if he wanted to keep his head. The yogi, however, coolly replied by explaining to Alexander that all he had power over was this body of his, which was going to drop one day. 'Whether you kill it now, or it dies a few years later on its own, so be it,' the yogi said. 'My spirit, however, is eternal, indestructible and ever blissful. You have no power over that. And this is what I truly am. You, therefore, may do as you please, and so will I. Now stop disturbing my meditation,' and with this, the yogi closed his eyes again.

Apart from the shock of being refused by someone who was not even bothered to greet him properly, Alexander was also astonished to see the fearlessness and composure of this holy man. He had never met a man who had truly no fear of death, or his own well-being, like this yogi had. This made him wonder what the yogi knew that he didn't.

It made me wonder too, because even at an early age I had had enough experiences of how life can shake you, no matter how hard you try to tell yourself that everything will be okay, or that things will work out fine. When I was still very young my mother was diagnosed with cancer, and there were moments where even the doctors did not know whether or not she would survive the treatments. For children the strongest and most unshakable source of strength, support and security is their mother, and the very thought of my mother suffering or maybe not staying with us was almost inconceivable. At other times, it may have been the stress of maybe not having enough money to buy even the most basic things that our parents would try to hide from us because we were too young to understand, or even if we did, to do anything about it. The change of joining high school was accompanied by another change at home, as our parents shared with my brother and me that they would be getting divorced, and suddenly I saw my father only over the weekends, or even less. And these are just some of the examples of situations that really shook me, or the people around me, and made me wonder how great masters like the saints and sages of the East that I had heard and read about had attained such lasting peace and mastery over their mind without having to rely on anything external, not even a home. This is probably why the stories of great saints of the past, or a documentary on TV about Shaolin Monks, or stories from my father about the yogis of India and Tibet that he had come across during his travels there, or the little Buddha statue that my mother had in her room had such a strong pull on me, as if silently calling out to me to learn more about their stories. What would I not give to be able to face life with such poise, feeling so calm and secure in any situation? How could people who had so little be so confident and peaceful, without relying on any of those things that we rely on for the same? It is this hidden strength and unshakable peace that has drawn me to the traditions of the East from a very early age.

Of course, this was nothing unique, as all of us in our childhood and school days have had to face challenges. Let's be honest, at that age those problems don't feel any less scary, difficult or important! Who has not had trouble sleeping soundly one time or another, knowing that when they wake up, they need to face an important math exam or presentation in front of a teacher who dislikes them? Who has not spent hours trying to gain the courage to ask someone out, facing an equally disturbed state of mind even after they have said yes, because what if things don't go as planned, or as they hoped? We start feeling we cannot live without something, and then desperately try to obtain it, only to find out that after that the stress and fear continue, because now we stand a chance of losing it again. If this is the case, then how to possibly remain peaceful in a scenario of such global uncertainty as what we faced during the Covid-19 lockdowns? The number of cases of depression, domestic violence, suicide and divorce increased drastically during this time, in just a matter of weeks! This only shows that we are not equipped to deal with uncertainty and change – or at least not sufficiently.

Yet, once in a while, you come across someone who seems to be unfazed by any of these things. It was the search for this unshakable peace that led me, initially, to practicing various martial arts as well as exploring some books and teachings of Buddhism and the Yogic traditions.

What is it that could make people so fearless, so calm, so comfortable, in almost any situation? I have met people who may have had very little, and yet they were happier than most people on this planet. Growing up with movies like *The Karate Kid* and *Star Wars*, I used to envy the boys who came across an actual 'Master' who could teach them how to master their mind and transcend it, giving them access to a level of tranquillity, power and centeredness that made them unshakable even when facing the most difficult situations or dangerous people.

The truth is, if we look back, we have also known a similar state in our own lives. If you retrace your steps to your early childhood, you will find a time when even you were freer and more peaceful. You were not bothered about how many friends you had, or whether they really liked you or not. You were not bothered about what you possessed, and whether it was enough for you. You were free, each moment, living life to the fullest. You were not worried about tomorrow, and you were not sad or upset about yesterday. Having a pebble or a twig to play with was enough to have a great time – for hours! Even if something would upset you, it would last for a matter of minutes at most, after which it was finished, gone, and you were onto the next adventure.

So then where did we go wrong? Where did we start conditioning our happiness and peace, our freedom and our security? Why did we start linking these to all those factors outside ourselves, be it our bank balance, comforts, relationships and success, that are often also outside our control? We have given away the control over our happiness and now it's time to take it back.

When we retrace our steps, they lead us back to ourselves, they lead us inward. We can only aspire to become unshakable, when we take ownership for our state of mind and how we feel about situations life hands out to us. This begins with coming to terms with our reality, with the world that we have created for ourselves.

Take an honest look at your life and think of all the conditions that you have created for your well-being, joy and peace. Knowing the problem and understanding it is the first step in finding a solution. Our securities are the things that we think give us stability in life, that we can fall back on. The problem is that we have a tendency to rely on things that can change any time, and then we get shaken. Our world falls apart. What is it that really disturbs you, scares you, or could throw you off balance? What is it that you cannot do without? And then inquire, why is that? What do those situations, conditions, relationships or comforts give you that you do not already have, or that you cannot do without? As a child we did not have any of these, and yet we were happy, peaceful, joyful, full of love and enthusiasm. So, what has changed?

If we look at our lives, we notice that everything changes, whether we like it or not. Some change may be slower, but that doesn't mean it isn't there. Look at your life closely. Your body has changed, and will continue to change, with every day, month, year and decade that you age. Your thoughts have changed, your likes, dislikes, your values and preferences. The music you were crazy about in high school may not appeal to you anymore, and the goals you have set for yourself would have also changed along the way. Your friend circle has changed, and the people you feel at home or comfortable with have changed as well. The way you see yourself has changed, and the way you want others to see you has also changed. Even your memory has changed – not just what you remember but even how you remember it. The same incident that broke your heart may have been difficult for you for some years, but after that, the feeling behind the memory faded. Some things that seemed unfair to you at that point in life are now remembered as a blessing in disguise, or a lesson that taught you how to become more skilful, or that gave you more depth and compassion for others.

If we look at our life closely, we have been experiencing change, and adapting to it from the day we were born. Sure, that doesn't mean that we were always happy, and that we never faced challenges, or got upset, but we were able to keep moving, and we found our balance again.

And if we look at our life even more closely, we will find that the very reason that we are able to perceive all these changes is because there is one thing that has not changed throughout. To notice change, after all, you need a reference point; you need one thing that stays the same, looking at which you notice that everything else has changed. That reference point is what you truly are. Your 'self' or 'being' or whatever you would like to call it. You.

Not your body, because you know that you are more

than just the body. The very fact that we refer to it as 'my body' and not 'me' already indicates that you are something separate from it. In the same way, we talk about 'my mind', 'my thoughts', 'my memories', and 'my feelings'. You may have never realized it, but on a subtle level you already know that you are something that is beyond all these different layers or dimensions of your existence. You sometimes get a glimpse of this when you meet an old friend, colleague or distant relative after many years. You are shocked – they have changed so much! You can hardly recognize them, and yet, you feel you are still the same, that you haven't changed. Even looking back at your own life, your early childhood, your primary and then secondary school days, looking at the pictures and remembering all the ups and down, challenges and adventures, you feel that even though life was so different, and even though you were so different, there is a part of you that has stayed the same throughout. That is You. That is what you truly are. And whatever happened to you, be it good or bad, has left that part of you unchanged. To become truly happy, peaceful and successful in life, we need to become unshakable, at least to some extent, and this starts by shifting our attention to that which does not change. To find that anchor in your life, that will allow you to sail through all the storms of emotions and challenges successfully, and that is this centre of your existence.

Tapping into this part of yourself, experiencing it consciously, identifying with it, is what meditation is all about. Peeling back the layers of our identity and existence, until we reach the point that is beyond time, and thus untouched by it. This is the source of your true strength, and to find it, we must look inward. Here I would like to add that meditation is not just mindfulness, it is much more, and we will discuss this later in the book. It is also not something that you can do by just downloading any app and listening to it when you have some idle time. It will require practice, some introspection and commitment – but don't worry, this book will guide you on this journey, and it is a path that is suited for all, not only those with a super fit body or an inclination towards leaving everything for a cave in the Himalayas.

Sure, it may have taken Kung Fu Panda or Luke Skywalker only a few hours to learn to look inward, find their true strength, and by doing so, become able to endure and even overcome the challenges they had to face, and it may not be as easy in reality. You and I may need a little more than a few hours to master this art, but that does not mean it is out of reach. And it is worth it, for everyone.

I had the good fortune to meet a true meditation master when I was sixteen, Gurudev Sri Sri Ravi Shankar, and since then I started learning about meditation from him. After receiving his blessings I have been teaching people how to manage their mind and how to meditate for fifteen years now, and if there is one thing that all my students have in common: it is that they are just like you and me. They may be heads of state, homemakers, university students, prison inmates, corporate executives or villagers – they all have similar problems. When they are stressed, anxious, or upset, they cannot enjoy their lives, they are not effective in their work, and they struggle to find their balance again whenever life does not work out as planned. Even the prospect of the possibility that things don't work out the way they hoped can be enough to cause sleepless nights, stress and anxiety. It takes away their ability to enjoy the things their lives had to offer, be it small pleasures or big achievements.

Haven't we all experienced that the tasty food or the beautiful scenery in front of us just loses its charm when we are stressed or upset or anxious? The quality of our lives is greatly dependent on the quality of our state of mind, and yet we have never learned how this mind really works or how to manage it.

In the next few chapters, we will embark on a beautiful journey inward, tracing back our steps to find out where we took a wrong turn or missed some of the signs. And know that you have already taken the most important step: you stopped. You stopped moving further away from that true happiness, peace and freedom that kept escaping you till now. By stopping, you moved one step closer to your goal. This is a journey that will allow you to start taking back control of your own happiness, one step at a time.

The more you progress, the more you will be inspired to start implementing the simple tools that you will be learning into your daily life, allowing you to not only become a happier person, but also a lighthouse and refuge for the people around you. Don't worry, this does not require you to sit in a lotus posture or exchange your comfortable apartment for a rugged cave in the mountains somewhere. You have been running around chasing things in this world long enough now. You may have changed jobs, relationships, cities or even countries. It has left you tired, and without any lasting result. The time has come now to rest, recharge, and to finally start looking inwards.

Wisdom Sutras

- The only constant of life is change. Acknowledge that change is inevitable and embrace it willingly.
- You experience the changes in the world around you because there is a part of you that does not change. Acknowledge the part of you that is unchanging and know that that is what you truly are.

10-Minute Exercise

Make a list of all the things that you rely on in your life that you cannot or would not want to do without and see how many of them are subject to change and could change any time. They could be the job you have had for the last ten years, the money you saved for your children's education, your relationship, or your own home that you will finally purchase after a few more years of doing the right investments.

The more you feel you cannot manage without these, the more you have conditioned your happiness, sense of security and freedom. Ask yourself why you cannot do without them – what is it that you are looking for outside yourself to make you feel comfortable or at peace? What is it that these things will give you, that you do not already have, to feel free in your life? Could you be happy without getting these as well?

2

Understanding How Our Minds React to Change

It was a warm sunny day – definitely not a day to be sitting inside, I thought. The summer holidays were around the corner, and with it the promise of freedom. The only thing that stood between me and a whole new chapter of my life were the high school final exams, and even though I was a bright student, we all have those few subjects that are challenging. Physics was the main one, and even though I liked the subject, my average scores throughout the year were such that I could not afford to mess up the final exam. Not if I wanted to graduate from high school at least.

I had been studying hard for the last few days, trying to squeeze as much information as possible into my brain, but unfortunately my mind worked the same as everyone else's: the tenser you get, the less you actually absorb. Studying for two-three hours straight, therefore, mainly consisted of worrying about the outcome of the exam, creating various scenarios of success and failure in my mind, and re-counting the pages that I still had left to study. Whenever I turned a page, one of two things would happen: a page with big diagrams, pictures or drawings would boost my enthusiasm as it had only little text to cover, while a page filled with nothing but text would mean a lot more work and tension. 'Come on, concentrate, focus, you have only one day left before the exam,' I told myself. But wanting to focus and actually doing it are, unfortunately, not the same, and it is not as easy.

'You have three hours to complete the exam. Please maintain silence and switch off your phones. You may only leave the hall after submitting your papers,' the teacher facilitating the exam announced. I carefully placed my watch, pencils, pens and an eraser on the desk. After an assistant had placed the exam papers on my desk, face down, I quietly prayed to whoever may be listening to help me through this successfully.

I took up the bundle of pages stapled together and turned them around. I quickly scanned through the questions, hoping to see many things that looked familiar or doable. However, I did not get far. The first two questions did not make any sense. Did we cover this? Did I miss this somehow? My brain was racing, trying to remember what these terms meant or when we had, maybe, covered this in class, but nothing surfaced. My hands became a little sweaty and I realized that I was left with only two choices. I could either panic, mess up the exam, and face the consequences later or

I could take a moment to calm my mind and see how I could still make the best of whatever life had put in front of me.

I closed my eyes for a moment, took a few deep breaths, and then decided to start from the third question, doing my best to answer them well. If I had time in the end, I could always come back to the first two questions, and maybe by then I would get an idea of how to solve those as well.

Unfortunately, this is a situation that all of us have to face in life at one point or another. The bad news is that it doesn't happen once or twice but is a cycle that just doesn't seem to end. No matter how well prepared you think you are, life has a way of coming at us in new and impossible ways that even the brightest mind could never have imagined. Things don't go as planned and the only thing you can do is manage the situation as well as you can. But here is the problem: we have never learned how to manage it. We have gone to school for so many years, and yet nobody bothered to teach us how to manage our mind. Or maybe, they also never learned in the first place?

From the early years of going to school the teachers would have told you, at least occasionally, to pay attention. It is not that you did not want to. Which student would not rather really focus, do well in school, and spend only one-third of the time on their studies and homework than we normally do? Which employee would not rather really concentrate on their work, so that they get more done with fewer mistakes, and that too in much less time? Would it not be so much easier if you could focus fully on what you are doing, rather than worry about what may or may not happen, or feel upset about something that did not go as you had planned? And yet, in all those years we spent on our education, nobody ever taught us how our mind, that which we use to study and do everything else in life, really works. We put so much effort yet, at the end of the day, we find ourselves at the mercy of this unpredictable thing called our mind. It can suddenly go for a toss, get stressed, sad or anxious, leaving us in a mess despite all the good things we have going for us.

You may have a good job, a nice family, and many of the other things you were once hoping for, and yet you find it difficult to fall asleep at night, no matter how many times you keep telling yourself that there is no need to worry about the presentation that you need to give tomorrow. No matter how sincerely you tell your close friend that she should just forget about that ex-boyfriend who dumped her, because you all agree that she is much better off without him, deep down inside we all know it is not that easy. She also feels that she should just forget about him, move on, be happy and enjoy life again, but how to actually do it? You can keep telling your mind to just drop it, but most of the time it doesn't listen to you – at all! This is exactly why so called 'positive thinking' or too much stressing on 'trying to be mindful' doesn't work at all – rather it can compound your stress and make you mentally tired.

Now what if I told you that this unpredictable thing is

actually not unpredictable at all? What if I told you that there are laws that govern our mind – fixed principles – which when understood properly can allow us to manage our mind much more effectively? If you look at your life closely, you will find that this mind of yours may actually be the biggest obstacle to you living a happy and peaceful life.

We spend so much of our time and energy trying to get all those things that we deem necessary to feel happy; be it relationships, a comfortable lifestyle, success, seeing the world, doing service, or something else. And yet, we find that even if we are able to get all that we desire, there is no guarantee that we will be able to enjoy it. A phone call, a text message, some unexpected news or an argument with a loved one can be sufficient to spoil our state of mind, and with it, the quality of our life. Many people living in the most beautiful houses, boasting lifestyles that so many are trying to achieve, are taking medication for depression and stress, and have difficulty sleeping peacefully at night. We need to wake up and realize that comfort and happiness are not the same thing, and that to really be content in life, we need to start looking inward. And when you do, the first thing you will come across is your mind.

The mind is without a doubt the most overused and under-utilized part of our existence. It literally plays a role in everything we do in life, and yet we have never taken out the time to really get to understand it. It is both responsible for our most creative and genius insights, as well as our biggest mistakes and failures. And yet, we have never learned how to manage our mind, or how it works. Learning to understand the mind, and the laws that govern it, we can finally start taking back control – over our mind, and thus, over our life.

If you observe your mind closely, you will notice it has an issue in just being with what you are doing at that point in time. It keeps running around, whether it is into the past or into the future. Just pause for a moment and observe it. While reading this chapter, you may have remembered some pending work that you still need to do today, or you may have been daydreaming about a different you in the near future, free from stress, worry and insecurity. So many past events or people would have come up, and all without taking any prior permission. The interesting thing is that our mind hardly spends any time in the present moment and we're often not even aware of this tendency. It is only when you make a mistake, like pouring some hot water over your hand when making a cup of tea or hitting your toe against the side of the coffee table that you realize 'your mind was not fully there'. It is because our mind is not on what we are actually doing that we make mistakes, do half-hearted jobs, and get mediocre results in life – not just at work, but also in our relationships.

If you examine yourself closely whenever you are focused, relaxed, happy or creative, you will find that these are the moments that your mind is fully in the present moment. Happiness, therefore, is a mind that is present, fully. And whenever you are sad, angry, upset or annoyed, you will find that it is because your mind got stuck with an event of the past – something that has happened, and that you are not able to let go of. Worry, anxiety and stress, on the other hand, are all signs of a mind that got stuck in the future – resisting a possible outcome of what is happening right now, based on your past experiences and knowledge. But we have all known a time when we were not troubled by our own mind like this. We have all experienced what it is like to be truly free.

Do you remember what it was like when you were a child? How free and happy and peaceful your life was then? You would wake up in the morning, full of life and enthusiasm. It was a new day, and you could not wait to start playing again. You were not worried about what would happen later that day, or how things would be tomorrow, or next week. Nor were you thinking about what happened yesterday, what that other boy said to you, or why that girl had not returned your toy. You were fully with what is happening right now in whatever you did. Even if you got angry or upset during the day, it would only be there for a moment, expressing it totally, and then you were fine again. You were so free, so happy, and so present. But when growing up, our life became more complicated, and so did our mind.

Nobody enjoys worrying about their future nor does anyone voluntarily dwell on their past experiences. The problem is that our mind does not listen to us, or rather, it often seems to have something against us. The more you try to stop thinking about a person, the more they keep coming to mind, and the harder you try to remember something, the slighter the chance of it actually coming back to you. The moment you drop the effort, you'll find that it suddenly reappears, almost as if to rub it in your face how futile your efforts were in trying to remember it. How many have not wondered if maybe God had something against them when walking out of an examination hall in high school or college, having struggled to remember all that they had studied in the previous days, only to find that those things that were right at the tip of their tongue, but just outside their reach, suddenly reappear in their mind's eye in all their glory, the moment they stepped through the door into the hallway? This is but one of many more classic examples of us having failed to understand how the mind works and how we fail to manage it. It is not that you did not study properly, nor is it that you did not know the subject, but you were not able to access it at the required time, despite all your sincere efforts.

Or was it maybe *because* of those sincere efforts? One more law of the mind is that it is governed by effortlessness, and not effort. The law of our body is effort, so this is what we are used to and have been taught. To train the body, to make it stronger, more flexible, or more skilled, we need to put effort, practice and train. Whether it is sports, learning to play an instrument, or anything else, it requires practice, which is effort. Our mind, however, is governed by a very different law. Whether it is remembering something, being creative, being focused, or being at peace, effortlessness in the key.

One needs to learn to let go.

Of course, we already do this sometimes, knowingly or unknowingly, otherwise you would not be able to fall asleep at night. But to be able to be focused and relaxed at the same time needs proper guidance and practice, and this is what meditation is all about. Meditation is a special state of restful awareness, and with regular practice it teaches the mind to remain relaxed and at peace even amidst activity, making it much more effective and resilient.

Another law of our mind is that the quality of our state of mind and its resilience are also closely connected to our energy level. If you observe carefully, you will find that the same situation or event does not always disturb you or at least not as much. Sometimes it takes just a small thing to throw you off balance and to send your mind spiralling down into a series of negative emotions, while at other times the same thing doesn't really bother you and you just brush it off. Those days, or times, when you are already tired, a little low, and when your energy levels are down, it takes very little to disturb you, just look closely. And when your energy level is high, when you are well-rested, and energetic, you will find that the same thing doesn't bother you as much at all. So, taking care of your energy level will also help you in managing your mind and emotions.

Here it is also important to add that this dynamic works both ways; your state of mind affects your energy level as well. We have all experienced being busy all day long organizing a surprise party, a celebration or some other festive occasion, and yet you still feel great at the end of the day. Doing something you are really passionate about sometimes even appears to give you energy, rather than deplete it. At the same time, we have also experienced how draining it can be doing something that you really don't like or don't feel like doing. Even just sitting and worrying about something is sufficient to drain your energy, all you need to do is just keep sitting and allow the mind to keep churning its way into misery. Even to become aware of the fact that your mind has taken a wrong turn you need a certain amount of awareness to have a chance to come out of it. This is why the yogis also practiced breathing techniques or pranayama in preparation of their meditation. Some of these techniques are effective tools to quickly energize the body and mind, making it calm and aware. They also used to make sure their diet and lifestyle were conducive to maintaining a high energy level, as they knew that all of these are factors that influence our mind as well.

The breathing techniques are actually one of the easiest ways to manage the mind and quickly bring it back to a peaceful state whenever it gets disturbed or loses focus. We teach a number of these techniques in the Art of Living courses, and it is one of the main things that made me join one of these courses many years ago during my high school days in the first place. I had already learned a little about using the breath to calm and focus the mind during my martial arts training over the years, but the practical application and use was very limited in our classes, and I was keen to explore this more and go a little deeper. The mind may be very difficult to manage and not really listen to you, as we already saw, but through breath it becomes much easier.

A beautiful example that I learned in my first Art of Living course was that the mind is like a kite, and the breath is like the string. Without the string a kite will fly all over the place, depending on where the wind blows, but with the string you can control where it goes, how far and how high. I learned that whenever our state of mind or emotions change, the rhythm in the breath also changes, and that this works both ways. Of course, we had also learned to steady the mind by taking our attention to our breath in martial arts, but suddenly I realized that there are many layers to this practice. There are not just two modes of being peaceful or disturbed; there is a whole range of emotions and mental states, and each of them has their own corresponding rhythm in the breath. And by becoming aware of the breath, and consciously changing the way you breathe, you can actually change or reverse these modulations of the mind. When someone gets angry, their breath becomes faster and shallower, while someone who is emotional has a very shaky breath. When you are sad or worried your exhalation is more prominent, while when you are relaxed and happy it is the inhalation that is naturally deeper. I started experimenting with these techniques and realized that even just becoming aware of my breathing and consciously slowing it down and making it deeper whenever my mind would get disturbed, would already help me a little when faced with sudden challenges. I may not be able to get rid of all the stress and frustration or irritation immediately, but at least my mind would be a little more centred and aware, allowing me to not act too impulsively.

But even then, knowing all this, we see that some people are perfectly fine, while others end up so miserable, upset or disturbed in exactly the same situation. You may feel you are dealing with such difficult challenges in life, and yet you can find people facing the same or even worse, and they seem to hardly be affected by it. How is that possible, I used to wonder? Here an interesting story comes to mind that I heard many years ago that gave me a clue. It relates an incident that is said to have taken place in the life of the Buddha, that gives us a glimpse of how to free the mind from the unnecessary anger, sadness and regret that prevent us from being happy and peaceful right now, as well as how to deal with unpleasant situations.

The Buddha was staying in a beautiful garden just outside a town for a few days, and every day he would preach for some time, sharing his teachings with those who had come to listen to him. A businessman of the locality started noticing that every day his sons and some of their friends would disappear for a few hours to go and listen to the Buddha, and he became more and more annoyed. 'This so-called holy man is filling the heads of my sons with all kinds of nonsense, while they should be here, running the business,' he thought. 'Sitting there with their eyes closed will not earn them anything!'

Finally, he decided to voice his disapproval and went to where the Buddha was sitting and teaching. After reaching the place he made his way forward through the crowd and went straight towards the Buddha. Suddenly finding himself in front of him, and not knowing what to tell the saint, he ended up displaying his anger by spitting in the Buddha's face.

The disciples of the Buddha got upset and angry but seeing that the Buddha did not say anything and just smiled at the man, they were unsure of what to do. The man, seeing the Buddha smiling at him, was shaken and did not know how to react. Becoming uneasy, he quickly turned around and walked out of the gathering and back to his home.

That night, the man could not sleep. The smiling face of the Buddha was haunting him – it was the one reaction that he had not expected at all, and he was not sure what to make of it. Having calmed down, he realized that his behaviour was uncivilized and inappropriate, and that he had done the saint a great disrespect. Feeling guilty, he went back the next day and hesitantly approached the Buddha, until he finally stood in front of him once more. 'Oh, Great One, please pardon me for my behaviour yesterday, I don't know what came over me. Please forgive me for my ignorance and anger.'

The man now looked up at the Buddha, whose face still bore the same gentle smile. 'I cannot,' the Buddha replied. Hearing this not just surprised the man, but even the disciples of the Buddha. Their master was the embodiment of compassion, and yet he himself was not ready to forgive this man for his earlier rude behaviour? 'I cannot forgive you,' the Buddha continued with a smile, 'because you have not done anything wrong.'

'My lord, I think you don't recognize me,' the gentleman replied. 'I am the one who came here yesterday and spat on your face.'

'No, you are not,' the Buddha replied, 'You are not the same man that you were yesterday. Nor am I the same person as the one that was spat on yesterday. And as both of us are different people, how then can I forgive you? Who is there to forgive, and who is to be forgiven, and for what?'

This story is often shared as an example of how true compassion is to be practiced, but it also teaches us a way to free our mind of the unnecessary burden of past events that keep haunting us. It is a technique taught in the Yogic scriptures that the Buddha, who was also a yogi, knew as well. It is the fact that the more importance we give to events, the stronger the impressions become and the more they bother us by becoming returning thoughts.

Have you ever wondered why certain thoughts keep coming back, and others don't? Have you ever paid close attention to the things you remember and the things you don't? You may remember what someone said about you behind your back a few years ago, but you will not remember what you had for lunch even one or two weeks back, unless it was something unusual or a special occasion. You don't remember your lunch because it was not important to you. This is also the reason why most of us don't remember any of the dreams we have at night. We may wake up feeling anxious, angry, sad or very happy, but after the initial few moments of realizing that it was just a dream, the emotions usually subside within seconds. And a few hours later we normally don't even remember the dream at all.

A colleague of yours may have abused you in your dream, but by the time you meet them in real life, you don't even remember it, let alone hold it against them. If at all you remember it vaguely, you may even have a good laugh over it, telling them what they did to you in your dream. But if even a fraction of what transpired in your dream would have happened in 'real life', it could have spoiled your work relation, and maybe even your overall peace and wellbeing at the office for weeks, months or even years. The only difference here being how much importance you gave to the event.

One may argue that we cannot compare these two scenarios, because dreams are not 'real', but the principle discussed here definitely applies to our mind and is valid. Another example could be having a random person call you an idiot or shouting at you on the street while you are on your way home. You may not be too bothered about this, thinking that the person may have mistaken you for someone else, or maybe that they might be drunk. In most cases, you won't even remember the incident a few days down the line. Were that person someone in your family or at the workplace, however, then it would be a very different story. Why? Because we give it that much more importance. Trauma is that state where you are not able to let go of some experience, something you have seen, heard, or experienced and it keeps disturbing you. So, in some ways you could even say that until we are really able to let go of the past, we are all traumatised to some extent.

It is therefore not so much the challenges and situations that really disturb us and take away our peace of mind, it is the impressions they leave on us that continue to pull our mind back into the past, or push it into the future, making it swing between anger, sadness and disappointment on one side, and anxiety, stress and insecurity on the other. And this is where we find a clue to live a more happy and peaceful life. The more you start looking inward, you start realizing that it is not so much the world outside that is defining our happiness and peace of mind, it is the world we have created within us. It is the baggage that we have accumulated when growing up, whether these are bad experiences or just dreams and desires of how we think things should be, that weighs us down and does not allow us to be at peace wherever life is taking us.

Realizing this is the next step that you have taken, one step closer to the goal. You will now slowly start to see that in all your earnestness you were not lacking in effort or commitment, you were just looking for the wrong things, or rather, you were looking in the wrong place. Come, let us continue, don't stop here. You are now ready to start asking the right questions, that will eventually lead you to the right answers as well.

But just like any journey that is really worth it in life, don't forget to pause in between and look around. Many a time the most beautiful experiences and most precious discoveries are those that happen while you were actually looking for something else. Our mind has many secrets to disclose to those who pause to really listen.

Wisdom Sutras

- The law of the mind is effortlessness. The more peaceful and relaxed your mind is, the more powerful it becomes.
- On the level of the mind, less is more. The emptier your mind, the happier, more peaceful and freer you are.
- The more importance you give to events, the stronger the impressions become. Wake up to the transitory nature of things – this will free your mind.

10-Minute Exercise

Sit quietly and take a moment to look at today and the last few days. What are the things that keep your mind preoccupied amidst your activities? What are the things or people that you are bothered by, that you are upset about, that make you feel uneasy, or that cause you to worry? Write them all down, one below the other. Take your time to really introspect. If nothing much comes to mind, or you don't remember anything right now, then you can take the next day to observe your mind and whenever you catch it getting stuck with something, whether it is in the past or the future, make a note of it.

Now look at each of the things that you have written down, one by one, and ask yourself why you are giving this so much importance. You will notice that your anger, sadness, frustration with past events, as well as your worries and anxiety about the future, are based on the experiences and concepts that you have accumulated over the years.

Wake up and realize that the past is gone. Whatever has happened, or whatever someone said, or did to you, has come and gone. It is nothing more than a dream, and the only power it has over you right now is the power you give to it. The more you are able to let go of the past, the more you will free yourself from the emotions behind those events that keep disturbing the mind – and the freer you will be.

Now for a moment close your eyes and consciously drop your entire past. Drop everything; the good, the bad, the right and wrong. Drop your very identity, and everything you think you know about life and this world. Drop all your experiences. Feel as if you have just come into this world and you are like a blank page. You have no past, no plans for the future, no goals, worries or concepts about who you are or how things should be. Dropping the entire past, become aware how empty and peaceful your mind becomes and how free you are feeling right now.

3

What Are You Seeking?

It was only 8 pm so I had time to finally catch up on my pending emails. The past four days I had been busy conducting a yoga retreat in Rishikesh for a group of yoga enthusiasts from South America. I opened my laptop, logged into my email account, and saw there were fifty unread mails. Scanning through the names of senders, I noticed a familiar one: Shweta.

It must have been about two or three years ago that Shweta had written to me for the first time, on Facebook, asking me for some guidance and blessings. She had just lost her job in Dubai and on top of that the guy that she had been in a relationship with had also suddenly left her, just when she was hoping to finally get married. She was quite desperate to get married also because she was now in her early thirties and her parents were putting a lot of pressure on her. I had given her some guidance on how to deal with the situations and manage her mind. In the months that followed, life was a struggle for her, where a few more possible marriage proposals did not work out, and neither did the job applications she wrote to various companies. And then one day she wrote to me that her prayers had finally been answered. She had applied at a bank that had an opening for the job she had been wanting for years, and she had been accepted. On top of that she had also been introduced Vishal, who was working in the United States. They had been speaking on the phone, and he was very kind, considerate, humble and had great values. It was a perfect match. In the months that followed the families also came in agreement about the marriage, and the day she had been praying for came: She got married to a wonderful guy, and moved to the US, another thing she had been dreaming about. In the months that followed I just received one more email about how life was everything she had been wanting, and that she was so happy with how things had turned out.

But then after a few more months I started receiving emails again. Shweta now needed to find a job in the US and was worried about getting a job that she liked and that would pay well. On top of that she was yet to make new friends in the US, and she felt uncomfortable when her husband would spend time with his friends there. They were not her type of people and she did not enjoy spending time with them. She did not want to let him out of her sight, but he also wanted some time with his friends. They would end up having arguments about this, leaving her feeling scared that he might leave her, and that she would end up alone

again. Her insecurities and demands put more strain on the
relationship and she grew more anxious. She was accepted
with a big bank after applying for various job openings, but
it soon turned out that the job wasn't all that she had hoped.
She felt that it was not what she had pictured herself doing
in life. She would go to work and be miserable there, feeling
that this was not what she wanted. Of course, she was lucky,
she told me, because she was not sitting at home, she had
a good job, and received a good salary, which is more than
many other people in the world. She had received everything
she had prayed for, and yet, she was not really happy.

I paused for a moment, took a sip of the herbal tea in
front of me, and then started writing my reply.

What do you want in life? Why are you here? Even if you
have not yet reached the point of asking these fundamental
questions, you cannot escape making choices in life. And
more often than not, you realize only afterwards that you
may not have ended up where, or with what, you wanted.
That joy, fulfilment, peace, true happiness, or love that you
were trying to achieve so badly, keeps slipping through your
fingers, almost tangible, but just out of reach. The more
miserable we are, the louder these questions become. Yet
all those who have truly managed to achieve these goals,
at least to a great extent, will tell you the same thing – the
answer you were looking for and the thing you want most,
are the things that were always there and that can never be

lost. This realisation only comes when you start asking the right questions.

If I look at my friends from high school and university, I can safely say that most of them ended up doing something very different than what they had actually studied. This is not because they were not able to get the jobs that they were most qualified for; rather it is because they were not at all interested in choosing those jobs. They had realized that they would rather do something else.

It happens to so many of us; you start something, only to find out somewhere along the way that 'this is not really what you wanted' or expected. Sadly enough, most people end up living their life like this. They don't know exactly what they want, or what they are looking for, and this keeps leading to disappointment or frustration. It is like getting into a train, not knowing where you want to go. The train takes you somewhere, you get off, only to look around and realize that this is not where you wanted to land. You don't know exactly where you want to go, but you are certain that this is not the place. Sounds familiar?

You are looking for real happiness, lasting joy and true freedom, but you don't know where to find them or where to begin looking. You wake up one day and realize that the relationship you are in is not what you had hoped it would be, or that your job isn't what you had expected, and you are very sure that this is not how you want to spend the rest of your life. All you know is that this is not it.

Here some choose to let life get the better of them and they keep moving down the same road, even if disillusioned, knowing somewhere deep down that it is not taking them to where they wanted to go. But it is too late now to turn back; they have already spent so many years treading this path.

Some others, who are braver, or more adventurous, may choose to take that leap of faith and try a new path. They choose one of the many options that are supposed to lead them to real happiness, and then dedicate themselves to it whole-heartedly. Even this can be confusing though, because if we look at the advertisements and commercials that we are bombarded with from morning till night, literally anything from a special soap, deodorant, pack of instant noodles, luxury watch, or new sports model or all-terrain vehicle comes with a promise of real happiness, the perfect family life, or a sense of true freedom.

Somewhere during our childhood, we stopped just being happy in the moment with whatever was there and started postponing our happiness, linking it to anything that was not there yet. You saw your elder sibling getting ready to leave for their first day of high school, carrying a big bag with books, a calculator, and other things, and you thought 'Oh wow when I finally get to go to high school and have a bag like that, I will be really happy.' But when you were able to get those things that you promised yourself would make you happy, it would just take moments for your mind to latch on to the next thing – if I have *that*, I will be really happy. Be it the latest phone your friend just got, a date with that pretty boy or girl, or a visit to Europe.

I remember when baggy clothes became a new fashion

in The Netherlands during my early high school days. It was new, it was cool, and suddenly the clothes I had been wearing for the last year seemed at least two or three sizes too small for me – and I hadn't really grown that much. My parents had divorced two years earlier, and my brother and I were living with my mother. We were happy, but we never had a lot of money, and we were used to buying our clothes at second-hand stores. I had been saving some money that I earned with a newspaper round I used to do, and recently I had joined as a dishwasher and kitchen help in a local bistro on the weekends. I couldn't wait to buy some of those fashionably big trousers and the oversized hoodie and t-shirts that would complete the style. Oh, and don't forget the shoes, which were ideally DC's, that was the main brand that all the skaters wore. I had already gone to the main shops selling these types of clothes in our city – a few times actually. I would carefully check out the price tags and calculate how many more weekends I would need to work to be able to afford them. The shoes were the most expensive.

Finally, the day came, and neither the heavy rains nor the stormy weather could stop me. By the time I came back home and parked my bicycle in front of our yard, I was drenched. But my face was beaming! I was carrying three plastic bags with three new t-shirts, two hoodies, two XXL trousers, a new belt (to hold up those ridiculously oversized trousers) and finally, my new DC shoes! I remember my mother looking through the kitchen window, smiling to see her son so happy. She shared my joy and was the first one to tell me to try on my new clothes and show her how they looked on me. Looking back, I appreciate her even more, because the wise woman she was, she must have known that those clothes I had worked so hard for would only keep their charm for a limited time. That is exactly what happened. The first few days, maybe weeks, I wore them ever so proudly, feeling great about my fashion sense. But soon enough, my mind had already found the next thing to focus on. If I could get that new portable CD player my friend has, I'd be able to listen to music anywhere, even when riding to school on my bicycle. I had once more successfully postponed my happiness. And like this, it goes on and on. We end up looking in so many places that we forget to pay attention to the subtle clues that our mind and consciousness have left us to actually lead us to our goal.

If you look a little more closely at your life and your mind, you will notice something fascinating. Whenever you truly enjoy something, whenever you experience pleasure or happiness, you will find that your mind stops for a moment and turns inward. The mind that is normally so caught up with and lost in all the experiences of the senses, getting pulled in so many directions, suddenly stops moving outward and reverses. Think about it: What happens when you taste something really delicious? Let's say a special delicacy ice cream your friend brought over. You take a spoonful and put it in your mouth, and then what happens? For a moment your eyes close and you taste it fully. You take the experience in completely, and a sense of joy, satisfaction, peace wells up, even if just for a moment.

Whenever something tastes delicious, you naturally close your eyes for a moment to relish the experience. It brings you joy.

A similar thing happens when you smell something exquisite, like a wild rose or jasmine or a subtle perfume. When you breathe in the smell, your eyes automatically close for a moment and the mind stops, while you take in the experience as fully as you can. But is it you taking the experience in or is it the experience that is taking you inward? Whether it is you hearing something beautiful, like some music that stirs something inside of you, or the experience of touch, like the embrace or caress of a loved one, they all have a similar effect on us. We close our eyes for a moment, our mind goes inward and we experience that momentary joy or happiness or pleasure.

Unfortunately, this doesn't always happen and this is where we get another clue. You hear a song somewhere, and it makes you feel so good and happy, that you find out what it is called and you download the song or stream it. The thought behind you wanting to have it is that when you would hear it again, you would again experience the same joy or peace that you felt when you heard it earlier. More often than not, it doesn't have the exact same effect on you later on, when you listen to it again. The same goes for a movie you saw that made you so emotional or the amazing meal in that new restaurant. We find that doing the exact same thing does not give us the exact same result. This means that the joy or peace that we experienced earlier was not just because of that song, movie or amazing food; these were just a trigger at that point in time for you to go inward and experience the joy that was already there. These external stimuli don't always trigger the same emotion in you. Think about it: If it was the food that made you feel a certain way, it should have the same effect on you every time you eat it, but it does not.

How many times have you gone back to a place, or ordered the same special dish, or rented the same movie, hoping it would make you feel as great as you did the first time or some earlier time you experienced it, only to find that it did not live up to your expectations? If you have never paid close attention to this, start doing it now, as these are valuable lessons that life is teaching us every moment.

Another clue to solving this mystery is when you start asking why people enjoy scary things or suspense. Have you ever wondered about it? Why did you want to go inside the House of Horrors as a child when there was a fair in town? Why do people like to read horror books or watch scary movies and thrillers? Why would anyone want to feel uneasy or scared on purpose? It is the same reason why people enjoy riding on a rollercoaster or driving fast on a bike or go skydiving. What all of these experiences have in common is that for a moment the mind stops and it comes totally to the present moment. Just think about it. Our mind that is normally all the time going to the past and future, worrying about what may happen, and regretting or feeling upset about the past, suddenly comes to a standstill. The story or movie or experience is such that in that state of suspense the mind stops and is fully present. And when the mind is in the present, it is happy. This is the only reason why all these so-called scary experiences give you joy and make you feel good. They are a means to temporarily bring the mind to the present moment. Any experiences that bring your mind to the present, to the here and now, so totally, will therefore give you some amount of fleeting joy and happiness because happiness is only in the present. It is never in the past, nor in the future, it is only now. When you realize that this is your natural state, that you don't need anything outside of you to be happy, then all you need to do is to learn how to skilfully bring your mind back whenever it gets stuck in the past or the future, so that you can be in the present, and thus happier.

Using this principle, you can go one step further and apply it to activities that aren't as interesting as well. By applying your mind fully to what you are doing, you will start becoming more peaceful thereby enjoying the task at hand more. This is also one of the principles behind mindfulness. The more you are able to be fully immersed in what you are doing right now, the less your mind will wander into the past – which causes feelings of regret, sadness or anger – or the future, which brings with itself anxiety, worry or stress. On top of that, your productivity, awareness and quality of work will go up because it is mainly due to your mind drifting off that you are less efficient, effective and attentive. Another benefit of applying yourself fully to the task at hand is that it will not leave any space for regrets, as it is the thought that you could have or maybe should have done that little extra that allows for the feelings of regret to creep in in the first place. So, doing things and living life with a mind that is anchored in the present moment has so many profound benefits! This is why small children are so happy, joyful, enthusiastic and stress free.

For those of us who don't remember what it was like when you were a small child: Have you ever wondered how children do it? They can fall asleep in any position and sleep so deeply and peacefully without a care in the world. You may be dead tired and yet you have difficulty sleeping in your comfortable bed because of all the worry, stress, pending tasks that just don't seem to leave your thoughts. Your mind keeps racing. A small child wakes up in the morning and is so full of energy and enthusiasm without needing any reason for it. We, on the other hand, first need a cup of tea or coffee, in order to start our day. Why? Because somewhere along the way that enthusiasm that used to be our nature has now been overshadowed by our worries, desires and stress. When we were small our mind had not yet become so complicated, and so caught up with the past and the future. For a child, the mind is still naturally in the present moment, and that allows them to do anything fully and enjoy it. Just notice how intensely a small child can look at something; whether it is a flower, a toy or their finger. There is so much we can learn just by carefully observing small children – you would be amazed.

For most of us, however, we find ourselves in the opposite scenario. When our mind is disturbed, we are unable to enjoy things, even if life puts the tastiest food or most beautiful scenery in front of us. Unless we learn how to unwind our mind again and reconnect with our true nature, we can keep spending all our energy trying to find peace and happiness in life, but we may never succeed.

So, is it wrong then, you may ask, to strive for job satisfaction, for example? Well, that depends on how you look at it. The beauty is that if you are able to be satisfied, irrespective of what you are doing, you will also be satisfied doing your job. And that is something worth achieving. On the other hand, if you keep on changing or rejecting job opportunities because you are waiting for that perfect dream job, you are not being realistic, and honestly, also not very practical. After all, the purpose of a job is to earn money and to be able to support yourself and those dependent on you financially. If that's the case, you need to make this your main criteria and not whether it is all that you dreamed of doing with your life. If the main purpose of a job is that you enjoy it all the time, then it is not a job, but a hobby. This does not mean that you need to be miserable though because, like I said, it is possible to get real job satisfaction. But the key there is that you are already satisfied, irrespective of the job.

The same applies in many ways to relationships as well. You will find that the more contented and happier you already are, the more you are able to give to the relationship, and the more your love and support for the other becomes unconditional. This allows the relationship to flourish. However, if you are coming from a space of need, expecting the relationship to make you feel happy, peaceful and loved, or at least less lonely, then there are much bigger chances that you are in for a rollercoaster ride, and possibly a disaster. Because, as my Master once beautifully put it, the thing about love is that its nature is to give, not take. The more you demand love, the more you destroy it, and the same holds true for a relationship. Whether it is a good friend or a partner, you will find that the more they start demanding from you, from the relationship, and the more they ask you to prove or show your friendship or love towards them, the faster it will diminish. Even if you had a lot of love for them before, it would start shrivelling up until you come to a point where the only way to regain your peace is to move out of the relationship. It is not wrong to look for satisfaction, love, peace and true happiness; rather it is natural and totally normal. These are our very nature, and it is what life will keep propelling us towards, until we regain it one day. But if we hope to do so one day, we need to know where to look.

There is an interesting story that beautifully illustrates this dilemma of ours that I first heard when my Master related it to us one evening during a public discourse. It is one of the funny accounts of the eccentric thirteenth-century Sufi philosopher Mullah Nasiruddin, and it beautifully conveys the predicament we find ourselves in even today. The story goes as follows.

It was evening and the sun had already set, when a gentleman who was on his way home noticed Mullah Nasiruddin crawling around on the street on his hands and knees, frantically moving here and there under the light of a streetlamp right outside his own house. It appeared that he was looking for something.

'Mullah, what are you doing here outside at such an hour? Did you lose something?' the gentleman inquired.

'Yes, I am searching for my key, but I am not able to find it,' Mullah replied, sounding rather disturbed.

The man felt sorry for Mullah and decided to lend him a hand. 'Let me help you,' he said, and he also got onto his knees and started looking for the key together with Mullah. This went on for some time, but the lost key was nowhere to be found. Finally, the man sat up and turned to Mullah. 'Where exactly did you lose the key Mullah? Are you sure it was somewhere here? Do you remember where you dropped it?'

'Oh yes, I remember exactly where I lost the key,' Mullah replied, and pointing towards his house, he proclaimed: 'I lost it there, inside somewhere.'

The gentleman looked at him confused, quickly got up and with irritation in his voice asked the Mullah: 'But then why are we searching here out on the street?'

Mullah, however, calmly and in a matter-of-fact tone replied: 'Because it is very dark inside my house. I am searching here because there is more light.'

Now, before we judge Mullah, we must look at our own life closely, because many of us are really not that different from him, at least in this matter. We look for the key to our lasting joy, happiness and peace in so many places, but they are all 'outside' of us. The truth is, the key to our true happiness and peace has always been inside, and as a child, we still knew how to use it. Somewhere along the way though, many of us seem to have lost it – or maybe 'misplaced' is a more appropriate term. We have started placing our happiness in things, people and conditions outside of us, and thus also outside of our control. Now we are frantically searching everywhere for the key, changing jobs, relationships, places where we live and holiday destinations, forgetting where we lost the key in the first place.

Don't keep repeating the same mistake as Shweta, as like her, you will keep finding yourself feeling anxious and uncomfortable with life, either because you are not sure if the thing that you imagine will make you happy finally will be within your reach, or because you are so afraid to lose what you have already acquired. Too many people have lived their lives falling prey to regrets of the past, discomfort with the present, and worry about the future, losing out on the beauty that our life in this world has to offer us.

Come, you are tired of searching, it has become dark already and it is cold outside. Now that you know where you have lost the key, it is time to finally start looking in the right place. If you are really serious about regaining your inner peace, you need to start going inward.

Wisdom Sutras

- When your mind is fully in the present moment, it is naturally happy.
- True and lasting happiness can only be found within you, it is never outside of you.
- Know that whenever you think that something or someone will make you happy in the future, you have yourself postponed your happiness.

10-Minute Exercise

Choose any one of your daily chores or normal activities that is part of your routine, but this time do it with a total sense of newness.

Apply yourself fully and feel as if you are doing it for the first time.

Involve your mind as well – do not let it drift anywhere, don't multi-task. Don't let it go to the past or the future. It may be washing the dishes, taking a shower, sweeping the floor, preparing some sandwiches, or making the bed. Whenever the mind drifts off, bring it back to what you are doing, and do it as well and as perfectly as you can. Forget about all the times you have done this already in your life and forget about everything you think you know about it. Forget about whether it is important or not and forget about what you would gain from it or how it will benefit you. Just do it, giving it your complete attention, involving your mind fully in the process. You will find that the more you are able to do this, the more you will start enjoying it. You will start feeling more peaceful, and happier.

This is how you used to do every little thing as a small child, remember? You would pick up a spoon with such total attention, and just watch it hang there in your hand. Everything would be a game, and you would play it with such enthusiasm, without worrying about the outcome. And you were happy!

4

Finding Inner Peace

'Mary, can you keep an eye on the helpdesk counter for the next thirty minutes? I am going out for lunch.' Mary nodded and gave me a smile.

'Enjoy!'

Stepping out of the large public library building, I was greeted by a gentle warm breeze that carried traces of the smell of the delicacies being served by the various restaurants in the square nearby. In the Netherlands the days where you can comfortably step out without any sweater or coat on are precious, and therefore even more enjoyable.

The public library where I was working to earn some extra money before joining university was located in the heart of Haarlem city, and was surrounded by all the main shopping areas. Welcoming the summer sun on my face, I walked towards the nearby public square where many people were enjoying their lunch served by the bistros and cafeterias. I walked into a small Turkish bakery and was greeted by a friendly man who already knew what I was about to order.

'Two fresh Turkish baguettes and a spinach feta cheese roll?' he asked with a smile. 'Yes please, the usual,' I replied. I came here every day to buy 'the usual' for lunch – it was fresh, delicious, healthy and affordable, so why change a winning formula?

'Here you go. Just give me two euros, that's okay.'

'No, no, you don't have to give me a discount! It is already very cheap,' I objected. The gentleman smiled. 'Please, just take it. It is nice for us also to have someone walk in here every day who smiles and appreciates our work.' I reluctantly agreed to pay the reduced rate but appreciated their heartfelt gesture.

Walking back to the library, I could already smell the freshly baked bread in the paper bag that I was carrying. The bread was still warm, crispy on the outside, and inside it would be very soft. Fresh from the oven! I quickened my pace, and after entering the building went straight up to the employee area on the top floor. Filling a big mug with hot chocolate from the coffee machine, I now went to what was my usual spot during the summer days – a chair on the rooftop balcony.

Sitting there, in the sun, with the occasional warm breeze gently carrying with it the sounds and fragrances from the city centre below me, life was perfect for a moment. I closed my eyes, taking another bite from the freshly baked bread, really tasting it, and I felt a deep sense of contentment and *peace spread throughout my body and mind. Slowly opening my eyes again, I looked down at the thousands of people moving through the alleys below, buying so many things, eating so many things, drinking so many things, and it made me wonder. Why do we think we need so many things? We keep running, thinking that one day we will get everything that will make us happy, but does it ever happen?*

I took another bite of the bread that was so fresh and tasty that it did not even require anything to be added, neither butter nor cheese or jam. When a simple piece of bread and a mug of hot chocolate and the sun on my face could give me so much happiness and peace, then why would I even want to run after so many things? What was the need? And then it struck me – the less you need, the freer you are. Not sometime in the future, but right now.

God, or the Universe, must have a good sense of humour, as trying to find 'true happiness' has for many probably turned out to be one of the most frustrating endeavours. Millions across the world have put themselves through all kinds of ordeals, be it climbing snow-clad peaks, signing up for a local hot yoga class, joining a Buddhist Zen retreat, or doing a sweat lodge, and maybe even trying drugs, all in an attempt to achieve what Kung-Fu Panda managed to do within one-and-a-half hour: find inner peace. And this is where many make their first mistake, because the moment you leave the house looking for the keys you left on the dining table, your chances of finding them have already reduced drastically.

Of course, nowadays finding or regaining your inner peace has become a much hotter topic than it used to be fifty or hundred years ago. But maybe that is because we have moved further away from it. It is nothing new that people look for peace or happiness, they have been since millennia, but it does seem like our modern lifestyle is in some ways taking us further away from this goal. Have you noticed how many of the older generations, the grandmas and grandpas, used to have such a calm over them? Whether I look at my grandparents in the Netherlands, or some of the old people I have met during my travels in India and other parts of the world, I often noticed a kind of calm, peace and simplicity that is rarely found in the younger generations. People sometimes even used to make fun of them a little, joking how all they needed was their usual sandwich for lunch, a nice book, and a cup of coffee with a piece of cake late in the afternoon to keep them happy and content. And yet, if you really think about it, it is that same peace and contentment that we are looking for but are not able to gain with all our gadgets, big screen TVs, and trips around the world. Have we, in our endeavours to attain bigger and better happiness and peace, become so dissatisfied with our lives and moved so far away from our nature that nowadays you can even hear a nine-year-old child confidently state that she is depressed? A nine-year-old child!

It is almost as if the fact that life has been speeding up continuously and becoming more and more hectic, has also made us more acutely aware of the need to slow down and move inward. Where yoga was something that was frowned upon by many in the West and many other parts of the world, even as recently as fifty years ago, often associating it with scarcely clad individuals that prefer a bed of nails over a comfortable sofa, we now find the most successful corporate executives and movie stars proudly boasting about their personal yoga practices – and that too sometimes even more scarcely clad than those yogis of ancient times!

Any advertisement or commercial that tries to sell you their product or service, in an attempt to convince you that you are not just buying the product but also your much needed relaxation, inner peace and fulfilment, will more often than not show you a person sitting in a meditative posture, displaying a sense of calm that may have caused envy even in the Buddha had he not been enlightened.

And yet, we rarely slow down sufficiently to pause for a moment, look at our life, and inquire why this true sense of peace and happiness continues to elude us. We are in such a hurry to get to the future and achieve our goals that we keep running, at least mentally. When is the last time that you had a meal and only had your attention on what you were eating and how it tasted? One has to be very careful that in the effort of achieving lasting happiness or true freedom in the future, one doesn't spoil the present by turning every activity into another item on the to-do-list, leaving no time to actually be happy or enjoy things right now.

You are eating, but you are also talking to people, or planning the rest of the day, or replying to your pending messages on your phone, or watching the news on TV. Which is why after realizing that you finished an entire plate of food you wonder why you still feel hungry, or at least not satisfied. You then look for some snacks, or some dessert or a sweet, not realizing that the lack of satisfaction doesn't come from not eating enough, but from not actually tasting and enjoying the food.

The same principle can be applied to any other aspect of our lives. In our enthusiasm to multitask, we try to also multitask our relaxation, our enjoyment, and our peace, and it simply does not work. I remember an interesting story that I heard many years ago from my Master when he was teaching us about this principle, that beautifully brings our attention to this point.

There was a king who was quite spiritual, and his subjects thrived under his just rule. One day the king heard about a holy man living in the mountains somewhere in his kingdom. Whoever had gone to visit the saint had experienced such peace and joy in his company and was so touched by his presence that word had quickly spread throughout the entire kingdom. Learning about this, the king asked one of his ministers to go and find out what is so special about this saint, and what techniques he practices, what daily routine he follows and how he spends his time. The king had met many holy men and he was curious to know more about this saint, whom people described as an embodiment of peace and contentment. After all, even kings were striving to reach such a state, and it had so far remained outside his reach.

The minister left for the mountains and after taking directions from a nearby village, finally found the place where the holy man lived. He decided to quietly observe the man, hiding at a distance, so that he could make a proper report for the king. A few days passed like this, after which the minister decided to return to the palace. When asked by the king about the holy man, there was not much that he could tell him though.

'Your highness, I have secretly observed the saint for three days and three nights, but I was not able to observe anything special about him at all.'

'That is not possible, you must have not paid close attention,' the king replied.

'No, my king, I am telling the truth. I did not let him out of my sight even for a moment. All he did was get up in the morning, take a bath, have his breakfast, work in his garden for some time, have lunch, rest for a bit, go for an evening walk or attend to any visitors that had come, have dinner, sit outside his door for some time, and then go to sleep. The same thing would happen again the next day.'

The king realized that his wise minister must be speaking the truth, and yet, he was not satisfied. He had been doing various spiritual practices for many years now, and yet this profound state of peace had eluded him. There must be a special technique that the saint had discovered that had allowed him to attain this holy state. The king, therefore, decided to go and visit the saint himself in order to learn his secret. Arrangements were made and he left the palace the next morning.

Having arrived at the place where the holy man lived, the king also first hid himself in order to quietly and secretly observe the saint. He soon realized that it was exactly as his minister had described, and not noticing anything extraordinary, the king finally decided to approach the saint and request him to share his secrets with him. The king was given a warm welcome by the saint and was given a comfortable chair to sit on. Apologizing for the modesty of his dwelling, the saint then offered the king some tea made with herbs from his garden, and a little while later they were both sitting in front of the saint's cottage, drinking their tea.

Being in his presence, the king could not fail to notice the utter peace and tranquillity that the holy man radiated, and the gentle smile on his face testified to the joy and contentment that he was rich. The king put down his cup, and then respectfully asked the saint: 'Great Soul, please forgive me for being direct, but could I ask you a personal question?'

'Of course, I have nothing to hide or feel shy about. Please ask,' the holy man replied with a kind expression.

'I apologize. I had been observing you for some time before introducing myself, in an effort to find out what special practices you follow that allow you to obtain such an elevated state. I was not able to discern anything out of the ordinary though. And now, sitting here with you, talking to you, I am still not able to discover it. Could you enlighten me on the special techniques or practices that allow you to be so free, so joyful and so at peace? There seems to be no difference between what you do and what I do, and yet, this profound peace still eludes me.'

The saint carefully placed his teacup on the small table and looking up at the king with a lot of compassion, slowly started speaking. 'My dear King, you have not looked closely. There is a world of difference between what I do, and what you do, and in this lies the secret.'

'But,' the saint continued, 'as you have asked me in all sincerity, I will explain it to you. When I do my work, I do my work. When I have my lunch, I have my lunch. And when I drink my tea, I drink my tea.'

Looking at the puzzled face of the king, the saint continued with a smile. 'But, king, when you work, you are also thinking about the past, planning, worrying about the future. When you have your lunch, you are also thinking about the affairs of the kingdom and decisions you still need to take. And when you drink your tea, you are not just drinking your tea, you are still so busy. Did you understand?' The king nodded, realizing that he still had a long way to go. And while the king was thinking of how he could somehow make this a practice and add it to his daily routine, the saint smiled – he was just having his tea and enjoying it.

We have seen in the previous chapters how all the signs are pointing inwards, and how the things that we run after are nothing but a promise of happiness and not the real thing. We saw that whenever we experience happiness, peace or joy, it is because for a moment the mind has turned inward and is experiencing our true nature. And we saw that we have all experienced a state where this was freely accessible to us, in our early years at least. Finding, or achieving inner peace is therefore a process of realizing or slowing down, not of gaining or achieving. When you stop running after all the things that you promised yourself will make you more comfortable, you realize that you are already standing in the place where you were trying to reach. True peace and happiness are your nature, and you can never lose them. You may not be able to perceive or experience it due to all the dust and clutter that has covered it, but it was never truly lost. In this way we are like an atom: the centre or core is positive, and any stress or negativity (the electrons) are only present in the circumference – only on the surface.

Any psychologist that says that deep down in you there is sorrow, anger or regret, has just not dug deep enough. They have only been scratching the surface. When you dive deeper, you will find that deep down inside there is only joy, peace, and enthusiasm. So, all you need to do is wipe off the dust and dirt of the diamond that you are. A diamond may get dirty, covered by mud, but it never ceases to be a diamond. It may have been in the gutter for a century, but the moment you wipe it clean, it will shine as brilliantly as it did a hundred years ago. And wiping off the dust, clearing the cobwebs, and opening the windows to let the fresh air in, is what meditation is. I would therefore put it like this: Meditation does not help you gain peace or happiness; rather it helps you to regain it, or give you access to what was already there within.

Our mind gets so caught up with all the impressions, concepts, expectations, cravings and aversions, because it latches on to them effortlessly, but we have never taught it how to let go of these again. As a small child this was not yet a problem but as the mind and intellect matured, there came a need to also know how to let go of experiences again because we started holding on to them.

Meditation is teaching your mind to let go and to anchor itself in the present moment, effortlessly. The more you are able to drop unnecessary past impressions and worries about the future, and the more you are able to be with what is happening right now, the more you will start to experience that true peace that is your nature – your inner peace. It is a state that can be available to you at any time, and irrespective of the situations around you, and this is what makes it worth striving for.

Meditation is giving deep rest to the mind, allowing it to find its centre, recharge and rejuvenate. Because our mind gets overexposed to so many impressions, and in an effort to get some relief we expose it to even more. This is mainly because we have never learned how to really give rest to the mind. It is like not knowing how to turn off the radio that you are tired of listening to, so to not have to hear it for some time, you turn on the TV at an even higher volume.

To relax you do different things to 'escape' from the continuous chatter in your mind – the worries and plans and desires – and yet it does not really recharge or refresh the mind, rather it just distracts it. Whether it is watching TV, listening to music, playing computer games, getting drunk or engaging the mind in any other way to keep it busy enough not to worry for some time; it does not actually give you rest or lasting relief – not at all. Our mind ends up in such an overworked state that even in sleep, it does not fully settle. The quality of your sleep suffers, and you end up having so many dreams and thoughts during the night that on waking up in the morning you don't feel fresh or rested, even after eight hours of sleep. So many need some peppy music, a cup of tea or coffee, or even a Red Bull or some other stimulant to really get going again in the morning. But it was not always like that, remember?

As a child, you would sleep so deeply, and you would wake up feeling so fresh and rested, that you would jump out of your bed to start playing again. One of the main keys here is the ability to let go. Because when a child goes to sleep it surrenders totally, it lets go of everything. The ability to let go is a quality that comes with dispassion, and in today's world, more than ever, we need to cultivate some dispassion to balance all the passion that is being encouraged. My Master once beautifully said: 'Passion is like breathing in, dispassion is like breathing out, it is letting go. You need both in life to keep going.'

Dispassion is the ability to drop everything for a moment, and we all have this quality to some extent because otherwise, you would not be able to sleep at all at night. It is a state of not craving for anything in this world or the next, at least for a moment. Unless you 'let go' of whatever is going on in your life, you will not be able to fall asleep at night. But doing so consciously can allow you to give real rest to your mind – a rest even deeper than sleep. And that is meditation.

Without dispassion, passion will turn into depression. Unfortunately, this is what we see so often nowadays. Depression is in a way a result of not knowing how to let go – of experiences, thoughts, events and desires. Even trauma in that way is a state where you are not able to let go of an experience. Looking at it in this way, many of us nowadays are 'traumatized' to some extent, because events and situations bother us so much that many need medication or therapy to sleep properly at night, to relax, and to deal with the situations that life throws at us. Excessive passion has been kindled in us for so many years, giving rise to so many desires, hopes, dreams and concepts, but we have not learned how to drop these again and come back to our centre. And if passion and dispassion don't go together, it gives rise to so many of these problems we are facing – be it stress, anxiety, depression or frustration. Dispassion is pausing for a moment and taking your attention from what is not yet there or what is still missing, to that which is already there, and knowing that you have all that you need in this moment. It is becoming okay with whatever is there right now, even if it is imperfect. It is in these moments that you experience true rest, peace and happiness.

Otherwise, even when we are happy for a moment, the mind will again start running, because then you start craving for the next thing, or worrying about wanting to feel like this forever, and not losing it in the future. It is only when you drop this desire of wanting to be happy and peaceful 'all the time', that you can be truly happy and peaceful and free. Otherwise, the desire to feel this way all the time becomes another stress, another worry.

Of course, dispassion also sometimes comes to us without our efforts, when we realize the impermanence of things. In ancient times they referred to this as *smashana vairagya* or the 'dispassion of the graveyard or cremation grounds'. I know people who experienced a drastic change in how they lived life, or looked at life, after being exposed to the sudden death of a near one, after surviving an accident or health problem that could have been fatal, or after getting to know that they only have limited time left to live. It opened their eyes to the truth of the impermanence of our life, causing them to suddenly start focusing on and appreciating what was really important for them, and not the usual small worries.

I remember once hearing an interesting story about this truth. A gentleman one day was able to gather all his courage and approach his spiritual master to ask him a question that had been there in his mind for years. 'Master, I would like to ask you something, but please promise me that you will answer me truthfully.'

The saint smiled, and looking a little surprised at the unusual condition added to the question, replied to the gentleman: 'Of course, haven't I always been truthful? I have nothing to hide, please ask.'

The man, hearing the encouraging words of his master,

decided to go ahead and ask him. 'Don't you ever get thoughts of anger, frustration, jealousy, lust or greed? Please tell me honestly master, how do you deal with these.'

The master looked the man in the eyes for a moment, and then smiled. 'I will give you your answer, as promised, but I will do so this Sunday. Is that okay?'

The man, having waited for years to finally ask this question, decided that a few more days also did not matter much and agreed. The next day the gentleman once more stopped by the Ashram of the saint to attend the daily afternoon discourse. After the program finished, however, the saint quickly walked up to the man, and gently taking him aside, spoke with a certain urgency in his voice. 'I am glad you have come today, there is something important I need to tell you.'

The man, perplexed, wondered what could be so urgent, as his master had never spoken to him in such a manner.

'In my meditation this morning my intuition showed me that you will leave this body tomorrow morning at six o'clock. I felt I should tell you right away, so at least you have some time to prepare yourself.'

The man looked at the saint with disbelief in his eyes, but then realized that the master had never spoken any untruth, nor had anything he had ever shared with them about future events not come to pass. Shocked by the news he had just received, he quickly went home, and gathering his thoughts, decided that he should make best use of the time he had left.

After writing his will and final wishes, he informed his

family and close friends, who immediately showed up and were heartbroken by the news. Sitting amidst all of them, some crying, some looking gloomy, the man decided that this was not how he wanted to spend his final moments and he told them that instead, he would rather spend his time cracking some jokes and remembering all the good times they had. And that's what they did. After spending some more time like this, he asked them all to leave as he wanted to spend some time by himself as well. They would all come back in the morning to see him off during his final moments.

The man then sat down by himself and thinking about what the future may hold after he would leave the body, he realized that if there truly were a heaven and hell, he would rather go to heaven. Figuring that he would rather be safe than sorry, he picked up the phone and started calling all the people with whom he was not on good terms, or whom he may have wronged. Apologizing and making peace with all of them made him feel at peace, as at least he had done all he could from his side.

Not seeing the point in sleeping away the last few hours on this earth, he decided to spend the rest of what was left of the night listening to his favourite music instead, and by the time morning came, his friends and family started arriving again.

When the clock showed 5:30, he lay down on his bed, ready to receive Death whenever He would come. At 5:45, however, the doorbell suddenly rang, and when one of his cousins opened the door, all were surprised to see the saintly figure of his master walk into the room. It is considered a great blessing to have one's master by one's side when leaving the body, as it is said this means you will be liberated, or at least you will go to the best possible place after death!

'Master, it is so compassionate of you to come all the way and be there for your disciple in his final moments, please take a seat,' the cousin said. 'Thank you,' the saint replied, and sitting down next to the bed the gentleman was lying on, he turned to face him.

'My dear child, I need to make a confession. I have done something wrong to you.' Before the saint could continue though, the gentleman interrupted him. 'Please, it doesn't matter now. I have found peace with everyone and I am feeling very contented and peaceful right now. I don't want to know. If you tell me it may stir up some negative feelings again, I prefer to die peacefully. I am happy.'

The saint smiled and then told him with a mischievous expression: 'But that is the point – you are not going to die!'

For a moment the man looked stunned, and then sitting up straight in his bed, looked at the saint and asked him: 'What do you mean?'

'My dear, I made up the story about the intuition I had in my meditation. You are not going to die – at least not any time soon!'

The man was not sure what to say, as this was all very confusing. But then the saint continued: 'But tell me one thing. During the last one day, did you have any thoughts of anger, lust, greed or jealousy?'

All of a sudden, the pieces of the puzzle fell into place, and the man looked up at the saint. 'Not a single one,

Master. I thought I was going to die; where was the time to be irritated with anyone or bothered by anything? It was pointless to waste any time and energy on that, all those things were so insignificant.' Smiling, the saint then said: 'Now do you have the answer to your question? I live my life as if every moment is my last.'

We all know that we are going to die one day, but we never truly realize what it means until one day we come face to face with the reality of this fact, and if that happens, it changes us. Until then we live as though we are going to live forever, postponing most of the things that matter to us, thinking we will do it some day later, and getting caught up with so many small things. We forget that the end can come at any time, and usually without prior intimation!

But when we realize that our time is truly limited, be it ten days or ten years or fifty years, we find that suddenly all those problems and issues that took up so much of our time and energy are so insignificant, that they are not even worth thinking about. Even this reminder, therefore, can help us come back to what is really important for us and how we want to spend our days. It can help us become more aware of the fact that the present moment is so much more valuable than the future, and at the same time it can help us to drop so many of the unnecessary worries, anger, hurt and jealousy, knowing that both we and the people we dislike, are going to die one day. So here the knowledge or awareness of the inevitable is not something that scares, depresses or stifles you, but it is something that actually makes you alive and free. We suddenly start doing the things that are really important to us – we suddenly start truly living our life. And it frees us from so many things that steal away our peace and happiness.

So many people keep living their lives hoping to one day find that inner peace, true happiness and real freedom that has been escaping them until now. But doing the same things and hoping for a different result is the classic definition of insanity. To get a different result, you will need to do something differently. Peace and freedom can only be found inside of you, and meditation helps us to settle the mind so that we can experience these deeper layers of our existence that lie beyond it. And here dispassion is an important and essential quality to develop. It is the skill to turn the mind that is all the time moving outward, running after so many things, inward, and bring it back to its source. Being able to feel comfortable with what *is* right now and knowing that you have all that you need to be happy and peaceful. When you really feel that you don't need anything right now, the mind immediately starts to settle down, and you start getting closer to your true nature. It is being comfortable with yourself, your life, and the world, however it may be this moment.

Many times, I am asked this question: 'How come you are so comfortable, so peaceful, just living out of a suitcase? Moving from place to place every few days. Don't you want a place for yourself? Don't you need some savings? What will you do when you get old? What if you will not be comfortable? Don't you sometimes want to take time off, go for a holiday? Or go somewhere else? It must be very difficult.'

Now how to explain to people that it is actually the opposite? How do I explain that the less you need, the happier and more comfortable you are? This ability to be comfortable anywhere, to live consciously but without worry, and to be happy with very little – truly happy – is available to all of us. You have no idea how beautiful life can be. The small joys become so big. True inner peace is so solid only because it is not dependent on anything outside of you. And this is what dispassion can bring to your life. Dispassion does not mean that you cannot enjoy anything, rather, it will allow you to enjoy everything. It can bring a beautiful shift in your life where you don't need to do anything hoping that it will make you happy, but instead, you can do those things happily. As my Master so beautifully puts it: this is where you stop living your life as a pursuit of happiness, and instead start living it as an expression of happiness.

One of the most brilliant minds and greatest saints and philosophers of India, Adi Shankaracharya said it so beautifully so many centuries ago in his famous song *Bhaja Govindam*. He said, '*Kasya sukham na karoti viraga*,' which means 'what happiness will dispassion not give you?' Dispassion is so often misunderstood as a state of apathy, inertia or lack of joy. It is the opposite. True dispassion will give rise to such dynamism, such happiness and joy, such freedom, that nothing can take away – exactly because it is not dependent on anything; not anything outside of you at least. And meditation is the practice that leads you to the place inside where it can be found.

Wisdom Sutras

- The less you need, the less you have conditioned your happiness.
- You need a reason to be miserable. You don't need a reason to be happy. Happiness is your nature.
- True freedom lies in shifting from living life as a pursuit of happiness to living life as an expression of happiness.

10-Minute Exercise

Sit quietly and close your eyes for a moment. Think of all the things that are currently on your to-do list. All the things that you want to do, are trying to get done, and that are taking up most of your time and energy now, and in the coming days and weeks.

Open your eyes and write them down. Write down all the things that came to your mind, and keep adding to the list until you cannot think of anything else that you are currently worried about, trying to get done, or want to finish in the coming days or weeks. Also write all the things that are bothering you right now, or that you are worried about. It could be a misunderstanding with a friend or relative, or the insecurity of whether or not you will get a good evaluation at work next month, or anything else.

Now take another page, or make another column. We are going to make one more list, but this time we will do it differently.

Imagine for a moment that you have only one week

left to live. Take a moment to think about what the things are that you would like to do or finish in this last week. What is it that you would still like to do, how would you spend your time? Write all these things down in the second list or column.

Let's compare both the lists you have made. The more similar they are, the closer you are to truly living your life. How much time do you make to do the things that you want to do, that are important to you, and that matter? And how much time do you spend on things that somehow appeared very urgent or important, but that are not significant at all? How much of your time do you spend thinking or worrying about things that are actually not worth your time and energy at all? Knowing this, can you drop some of these things, and spend some more time doing the things that are really important to you?

5

Meditation:
Mindfulness . . . or Emptiness?

After travelling for a few hours, we finally reached our destination: A beautiful complex in the countryside of the Netherlands. I had been able to convince a few of my friends to join me on this four-day retreat where we would be learning about mind-management, breathing techniques and meditation. It was the first program for youth organized by the Art of Living in the Netherlands.

I had been practising various martial arts for years, and our Judo, Aikido and Ninpo Bujutsu classes would usually start with a few moments of deep breathing and quieting the mind, but I had been wanting to explore these practices more. Every once in a while, I would sit down in front of the big Buddha statue in my room that my uncle had brought back after one of his trips to India. I would look at the perfect posture and the serene expression on the face of the Buddha and finding a posture that was kind of similar but did not require as much flexibility as the ancient yogi possessed, I would close my eyes and try not to think of anything. The problem is, as we all know, that it is really not that simple. Reading a few books about Zen and meditation had only made things worse. My thirst for an authentic experience of real inner peace had increased and at the same time it had made me even more acutely aware of the fact that I would probably not be able to figure this out by myself. Having met the founder of the Art of Living, Gurudev Sri Sri Ravi Shankar at a large public program in Amsterdam a few months earlier, and experiencing a meditation guided by him during the program, I now felt I had finally found what I was looking for: An authentic path and a realized master that could lead me to my goal. When a few months later we got to know that the Art of Living would be organizing a residential foundation program for youth, where I could learn more about breathing techniques and meditation, my younger brother and I immediately signed up.

'Hi, my name is Claudio, you guys must be here for the All-Round Training in Excellence?' The English accent of the young gentleman gave away that he was either from Germany or maybe a country bordering it. It turned out he was from Switzerland and he was one of the first trainers in Europe that had been certified to conduct this new program.

'I will be leading the program,' he said with a smile. He must have been in his late twenties or early thirties, and with

his short hair and elegant style of clothes, he looked more 'cool' than 'Zen' to me. I had not really given a lot of thought to what to expect from a retreat like this, but upon meeting Claudio I realized that I had anticipated a little more incense and meditation bells. Not that I had any problem with those – I love the Eastern cultures and traditions – but meeting this cool young guy made me curious about what the program would be like.

In the days that followed, we explored all that had been advertised, and more. We learned more about how our mind works and how to manage it more effectively, we learned some breathing techniques to increase our energy level and relax the mind, and we had our first experiences with meditation. This is where I learned one of the most valuable and important principles of true meditation: It is the 'art of letting go'.

For years I had been trying to focus my mind into that state of total tranquillity, as 'mindfulness' and awareness and focus were all an essential part of many of the things I had experienced and read about, be it my martial arts classes or the books on Zen. It was only now that I realized that focus or mindfulness is only the first step, it is preparation. Real meditation, that state of deep rest and unwinding of the mind, only happens when you let go. And this is easier said than done – it needs the right guidance, and some practice, to really get it right. But the results were obvious.

Looking at Claudio's face sitting across the big wooden table during our lunch on the third day of the program, I couldn't help but ask, 'How come you are always smiling?' It had struck me multiple times during the last few days that he was smiling almost all the time. Not an exaggerated or unnatural type of grin, but a very subtle, contented type of smile, as if he was really enjoying every moment. Something very unusual for an adult, especially in today's hectic world.

Claudio looked at me, smiling even more now, and putting down his sandwich said, 'Oh, that is because I practice the breathing techniques and meditation every morning without missing a day. I have been doing so for the last few years already. You try it for yourself when you go back home. It really works!' He took a sip of his herbal tea and picked up his sandwich again.

He may have been very casual about the whole thing, but he didn't fool me. I may have been only a teenager at that point, but I had already seen enough of the world to know that such peace and happiness are not that easily achieved – at least not by many people that I knew. Could meditation really be this effective?

Nowadays meditation is quickly going down the road that yoga has travelled as well in recent years. Almost everybody has heard about it and many think they know what it is all about. In a matter of decades yoga and meditation have seen a huge transformation – be it in branding, image and association, as well as the range of practices and concepts associated with it. Where in earlier days a true yogi was often pictured to be a scarcely clad skinny man sitting on a bed of nails or standing on one leg, some of the most famous icons of yoga are now scarcely clad skinny women sitting on a beach or standing on a mountain on one leg. Okay, fair enough, the scarcely clad, skinny and the one leg still remain, but the loincloth and the yogi that was more of an outcast than a part of mainstream society have successfully made way for designer outfits that are sometimes not too different from a bikini, and the successful and sought-after corporate trainer or wellness coach.

Meditation, sometimes being a part of yoga practices as well, has evolved along with it, and in the process a lot of its essence has been lost, while some other elements were added. In an effort to make it more 'secular' and even easier to market the term 'mindfulness' became popular, almost as if it was a miracle solution that finally stripped meditation of the cultural baggage that was weighing it down. Mindfulness became another – and more preferred – word for meditation, and some of its most essential aspects were forgotten, or deliberately brushed aside.

So, before we embark on our journey of discovering the treasure that is meditation, let us first clear some of the jungle that has covered it and understand a little better what it is, and what it is not. Because nowadays it has become like yoga: everybody knows it, without actually knowing it, leading to people often discarding it without actually experiencing it, while thinking they have. And nothing is worse than someone giving up on meditation even before they have had an authentic experience, as it means their misconception has deprived them of the many wonderful benefits that meditation has to offer. Too many times I have come across people who told me that meditation does not work for them, only to find out that they had at some point given mindfulness a try, and it had not given them the desired results or even left them more frustrated.

One of the best explanations of the difference between meditation and mindfulness as it is usually practised nowadays was given by my Master when he was interviewed by Vishen Lakhiani, the well-known CEO of Mindvalley, an online learning platform. The special session was part of a big international conference in Bengaluru organized by the Art of Living that saw many distinguished leaders in their respective fields, be it various industries or government from all over the world and I was fortunate to be present there as well.

When Vishen asked Gurudev Sri Sri Ravi Shankar about meditation becoming more popular in the West as mindfulness, and his thoughts on the same, he beautifully replied: 'Mindfulness is not (the same as) meditation. Mindfulness is like the driveway, it is like the balcony or portico of the house, but there is so much more beyond that, beyond mindfulness. The real house lies beyond that.' Mindfulness can get you into the garage but sitting in the garage is not the same as sitting in your living room.

Mindfulness practices are basically all about making an effort to be fully with what you are doing, or what is happening, at that very moment. It is about becoming aware, or 'mindful', of what is happening right now. This may sound simple, or very natural, but unfortunately our modern lifestyles and society have conditioned us to multitask almost anything we do, including thinking and paying attention.

While having breakfast you are watching the news on TV, while at the same time also scanning through the emails on your phone to see if anything important came in last night. And because you are sitting at the same table at the same time as some of the other family members, it can also be classified as 'family time', so you save some time there as well. Even when doing simple actions like making coffee or taking a shower, our mind is simultaneously planning, worrying, and so much more. This is where mindfulness becomes beneficial.

When we start to look at our mind, we realize the mess it is in, and doing things consciously, with attention and awareness, becomes a practice to consolidate and slow down the mind. We are training the mind to become less scattered again, more focused, and thus more in the present moment. It is like consciously making an effort to eat fresh and healthy food again, like fruits and vegetables, because our modern lifestyle has made us so habituated to having 'junk' food. It's sad, maybe even alarming, that in today's world it may often require extra effort, and sometimes even extra expenditure, to eat healthier and natural food that was the common staple diet for all a century ago. But nobody else is to blame, as we have ourselves created the fast-food lifestyle, just like we created the mental overload of impressions that we are facing today. And this is where consciously going back to a more simple and natural way of life can already benefit us a lot, both when it comes to diet and when it comes to our mental activity.

Mindfulness can help us in settling the mind, slowing it down and creating more space and awareness to consciously observe the mind and all its tendencies and patterns. Reducing the overload of impressions that we tend to expose our mind to also has proven scientifically to have many benefits, such as reducing stress and anxiety and improving overall mental health. It can also help in observing one's thoughts more neutrally, without identifying too much with the thoughts that come up. But even though mindfulness in its original form in the ancient traditions was meant to do exactly all this, it was clearly taught as a step towards or preparation for meditation – it is not the same thing. And if you forget that, or don't know that, then you may miss out on the main course of the meal, so to speak. It is like sitting in your garage thinking it is your living room – it is not the same thing, and it will not give you the same experience. Nobody can really relax in the garage, for that you need to get out of your car and into your home.

Though mindfulness is in some ways a good place to start, it's often not an easy one, especially initially, because the mind is so active, and we have never learned how to properly relax it. For many, relaxing means maybe having a beer, or watching TV, or doing something else 'to take your mind off things', where 'things' refers to your issues, problems, stress, unfulfilled desires and worries. These activities don't relax the mind though, it just takes your attention off all the thoughts racing through your head, giving you a break from all the noise. So here mindfulness is doing the opposite: it is making you more acutely aware of all the noise – something which, for many, can be quite difficult to confront.

The truth is that, for many it is quite scary to just sit down, maybe even close their eyes, and then do nothing but observing their thoughts – because it is like opening a cupboard full of junk that you have consciously avoided during spring cleaning for many years. The moment you open it a little and the dust and stench comes out, there are suddenly many more reasons to just leave the thing closed and try and forget about it than actually opening it and start on trying to clean it out. Think about it. For someone who is really worried, stressed, agitated or afraid, the last thing that will make them relax or come back to their centre is sitting and doing nothing but thinking about or looking at that fear, worry or problem that is disturbing them.

Also, focusing on something for more than a few seconds is easier said than done – so here we see that even to practice mindfulness properly, you already need to have a certain amount of peace and mindfulness to begin with!

Trying to tell your mind to be quiet, or force it, is like trying to intellectually explain to a child why it is supposed to sit quietly. You can give all the arguments you want, but it is not going to have any effect on the tantrum in front of you – except maybe an adverse one. It is in the nature of the mind to be active, so rather than trying to wrestle with it, wisdom is to transcend it.

The main things that disturb us, even more than the thoughts, are actually the feelings behind them. More than the 'thought' of insecurity, it is the 'feeling' of insecurity that is bothering us. Despite trying to rationalize things and explaining to yourself that there is no reason to feel upset, annoyed, insecure or scared, you still end up feeling that way because feelings are subtler than thoughts, and thus more powerful. So, to really address our problem effectively and efficiently, we need to attend to levels of our consciousness that are even more nuanced than our thoughts – we need to transcend the logical mind and go inward even more. Just like with anything else, the crux here is learning *how* to do it.

Mindfulness may give you more insight into the chaos inside your head, the uneasiness you feel with certain people or a situation, or the challenges that you are facing in life, but it may not help in actually getting rid of those feelings or emotions because it doesn't take you beyond your mind to the source of peace, joy and stability. At least not until you are a very advanced practitioner. Inner peace is not an intellectual thing, it lies much deeper, even beyond the feeling level. For us to be able to access this, we need to be able to tap into deeper layers of our consciousness. Unless you are a very advanced practitioner, mindfulness still confines you to the thinking mind, you are still having thoughts, analysing them, observing them, and this is not allowing you to go deeper, and to 'switch off' the mind for some time, giving it some actual rest and 'cool down' time. Some may even end up engaging the mind even more, making the whole thing actually more tiring for the mind, and this can be another challenge if you practice mindfulness too much. There is the risk of losing your ability to relax and go beyond the mind – to just be with the unknown. I have come across several people who were struggling with this as they became so focused on being fully aware of what they were doing that it actually created another type of tension, where they found it difficult to simply relax the mind. They couldn't just sit and enjoy something as they were only focussed on observing themselves or their minds.

This is one of the things that can happen when spiritual practices or techniques that have been tried and tested and authenticated by thousands of years of tradition and scriptures that provide the supporting context and guidance, are taken out of that context and repackaged as a modern quick-fix solution, preferably without any reference to its original context.

Even the roots of most modern mindfulness practices, which lie in Buddhism, are part of a much broader system of practices and teachings. It includes many of the aspects of the yogic traditions and this is what the usual 'role models' of these practices have made their own, and these should not just be brushed aside. The Buddha practised many things and was an accomplished yogi. When he sat down under the Bodhi tree to meditate, he was not just doing a mindfulness exercise – he went into deep meditation and transcended the mind, attaining a state of deep samadhi, or equanimity beyond the mind.

Meditation is more than mindfulness, much more, and as such it also has so much more to offer. Thinking that a few minutes of mindfulness will get you there is foolishness, and it would be a shame if you never make it beyond your garage into your actual home. True mindfulness is actually a natural result of deep meditation – it happens naturally as a product, without all the effort and struggle that most of the modern-day mindfulness practices require.

Nowadays, the words mindfulness and meditation are often used interchangeably, and the word meditation nowadays usually refers to a whole range of different practices. But true meditation is going beyond the mind, to experience that state of 'no mind' or emptiness. It is in this space that the mind gets its deepest rest, even deeper than sleep, and where it can really refresh and recharge itself. It is the mind turning inward, going back to its source. It is the art of doing nothing, the art of letting go. And that is why if you look at the Zen tradition also, for example, the whole purpose of many of the practices is actually to go beyond the mind, snap out of it or transcend it, rather than to keep engaging and observing it, or trying to make it settle down. Zen Masters use all kinds of approaches to get their students to 'snap out of' the logical thinking mind, into the unknown pure 'being'. More advanced stages of mindfulness practice do take you to a more restful and calm state of mind, but even then, to get the deeper benefits that meditation offers, we have to transcend.

One of the big challenges is that even just one or two things that trouble or disturb you are sufficient to take away your peace of mind. It takes just one or two things to shake us, and that in turn affects the way we function, approach the situations that come in front of us, and interact with the people around us. Challenges will keep coming in life, but for us to become bulletproof or at least fairly resilient, we need to learn to deal with those situations that disturb us and go beyond them. Everything else in life can be perfect, and yet you find that that one problem or issue is sufficient to make you lose your sleep. There is an interesting story that my Master once shared with us that comes to mind here. It is said to relate an instance in the life of the Buddha and conveys a meaningful message.

A gentleman had been attending the sermons of the Buddha just outside his town when the Buddha and some of his disciples had decided to spend some time there while passing through the region. With each passing day, the man became more inspired by the teachings of the saint, and the ideals that his followers had dedicated their lives to. Finally, after attending one more sermon of the Buddha, the gentleman made an important decision. He planned to approach the Buddha with the request of being initiated as one of his monks. Having lived a good life, his family was taken care of and his children had all married and were well-settled. They had taken over the family business, which meant the man was free to retire whenever he felt like. Considering all this, the man felt that the time had now come to apply himself to making a difference in society, as well as to strive towards his spiritual advancement.

He went to the place where the Buddha was staying and humbly requested for audience with the Master. He was asked to wait for some time, and finally one of the disciples of the Buddha came to take him to where the Buddha was seated. Having bowed down, the man placed his heart's desire before the saint, asking him whether he would accept him as his disciple, and ordain him as a monk. Looking at the man for a moment, the Buddha answered: 'Your desire is a noble one, but we have one condition for anyone that wants to take up the life of a monk in our order. You need to be able to feel compassion for all the beings, which means you need to accept all as they are. Please take your time to consider this, and if you feel that you will be able to do this, come back tomorrow and I will initiate you.'

The man gratefully bowed down once more, and after going home found a place to sit quietly so that he could meditate on the words of the Master. He sincerely looked into his heart to see if he would be able to accept all. The next day arrived, and the man once more set out towards the place where the Buddha was staying. Having waited for a while, he was once more ushered in for an audience, and paying his respects to the Master, placed a flower at his feet.

'Have you looked into your heart?' asked the Buddha gently. 'Will you be able to accept all the way they are, and love all?'

The man looked up at the Master and replied in all honesty. 'I have given it a lot of thought Master, and I realized that I can accept all, yes, except for two people. What they have done to me and my family is very difficult to forgive, let alone forget.'

The Master looked at him with a lot of compassion and then replied slowly: 'Okay, I appreciate your honesty. In that case, we will make an exception for you. You don't need to accept all the people in order to be ordained as a monk here. You will only need to accept those two people.'

If we look at ourselves honestly, we will find that we are all a lot like that sincere gentleman. We don't have a lot of problems all the time, maybe just a few. But those one or two things are enough to shake us and spoil the quality of our life. A small thorn in your shoe can make walking so uncomfortable, and a small grain of sand is enough to blind your vision and irritate your eye. The true skill here is to be able to accept those two people that are disturbing our mind, it is only then that we can be truly peaceful and happy. And if you look at life closely, you will find that those two people or problems don't remain the same throughout – they keep changing. But time and again there will be these one or two things that can make it difficult to sleep peacefully at night, or that can stop you from feeling at ease. Just like with the thorn in your shoe or the grain of sand in your eye that pricks or irritates you more if you rub it, the more you resist or try to get rid of some unpleasant thoughts or feelings, the more it seems to gain strength and power over you. So here the key is effortlessness, not effort. Letting go, not struggling. This is meditation. This is the skill we need to learn.

Our mind is often so busy and overloaded with impressions nowadays that even our normal sleep isn't sufficient anymore to give all the rest to the mind that it needs. This is why even after sleeping for seven-eight hours, you still don't feel really fresh when you wake up because even at night we don't have the time to digest all the impressions we accumulated. This is one more reason we need meditation, as it gives much deeper rest than sleep, allowing the mind to settle much more. True meditation is restful alertness, where in just twenty minutes it can give our mind the same amount of rest that it would normally get in four to six hours of sleep. True rest comes through effortlessness, it can never come through effort. We saw earlier how the body and mind work according to different laws, and while the body requires you to put effort, the mind is most effective when approached through effortlessness. This principle holds all the truer when you want to relax the mind fully and go beyond it.

I have experienced so many times for myself, as well as in many programs that I have conducted, that in just a matter of fifteen minutes people often feel fresher, more energetic, more alive, more rested, more positive and more peaceful – just by doing a simple meditation practice. Observing your mind and thoughts for 15 minutes may slow down the mind a bit and give you some more clarity, but it rarely has such quick and powerful effects as a simple dip into the consciousness that lies beyond the mind –

even for beginners, or people that may have never tried any such practices.

Of course, here guidance makes a big difference, and in the following two chapters I will share many of the basic steps, tricks, dos and don'ts that I have picked up and experienced over the last two decades in my own personal practice under the guidance of my Master, as well as valuable learnings that I observed during the many programs that I have taught.

Consciously putting the mind to rest is meditation. When the mind and nervous system are able to unwind and let go of many of the unnecessary impressions, stresses and strains that we tend to accumulate, you will find that it is naturally more anchored in the present moment. But because it requires us to go beyond the mind, it is not something you can learn by just understanding it intellectually. It is a skill that comes with the right guidance, and sincere practice. Are you ready to start exploring the unknown?

Wisdom Sutras

- Meditation is not concentration or focus – it is the art of de-concentration or letting go.
- Effort can steady and focus the mind, but to transcend it you need effortlessness.

10-Minute Exercise

Sit quietly with your eyes closed in a place where you will not be disturbed. Find a position in which you are comfortable so that the body can relax. Take a few normal deep breaths in and out, and for a few moments keep your attention on the breath, observing it as it goes in and out of the body on its own, effortlessly.

Now become aware of your thoughts. Whether good thoughts or bad thoughts, do not resist, analyse or judge them. Just let them come and go on their own. You do not entertain or hold on to pleasant or positive thoughts, and you do not judge or resist any negative thoughts. Not giving any special attention to either, you are not analysing them, nor are you focusing on anything. Just remain there as a witness to your own mind and whatever is happening right now.

Let go of all effort and unwind.

Whenever you notice that your mind has started galloping on some or the other thought again, or if it has begun planning something, gently bring it back again to itself. Once more, take a gentle deep breath in and breathing out let go and relax in the here and now.

Do this for some time and then observe how you feel afterwards. With some practice, you will notice that the mind naturally feels fresher and becomes more aware and alert afterwards.

6

Starting Your Meditation Practice

When we walked out of the door, the first thing I saw was the majestic sight of the beautiful Table Mountain against a clear blue sky. It is one of the many things that makes Cape Town my favourite city in South Africa.

'We will have to squeeze a bit as I brought the truck,' Francois told us. 'I didn't expect that there would be three of us,' he apologized. Francois is a big guy, with an athletic build – he had been a professional model before he took up yoga and started various service projects in the poorer and more dangerous areas in and around Cape Town. Apart from the fact that he has a heart of gold, I was also happy for him to come along because the neighbourhood we were going to was one of the dodgier ones, and because he speaks fluent Afrikaans. This would come in handy as the man we were to meet spoke only Afrikaans, we had been told.

'Do you know the address?' Francois asked us. 'Yes, we

were able to speak to his wife and her son, and she explained it to us. We have to go to Delft.'

'Okay, I know how to get there. How did you even find out about this guy?'

'I happened to come across an article in the Washington Post *one or two months ago,' I replied. 'A friend who knew that I am now working in Africa had forwarded it to me.'*

The article had caught my attention as it related the story of Fredie Blom, a simple man living in this part of Cape Town, who was considered to be the oldest man alive. An official declaration of the Guinness World Records organization was pending, as these things often take time to verify, due to lack of proper records. But as per the records available, Fredie had turned 115 earlier in the year, and as I had just returned to Cape Town after many months, I did not want to miss the chance to meet this gentleman. We had been able to contact his wife and they had kindly agreed to receive us today. On their request, we also brought some groceries, including some of Fredie's favourite things.

Having finally turned into the narrow road where the small house was located, we parked the car and carried the box of groceries with us up to the porch. 'Good morning. You must be the people that called? Please come in.'

We were welcomed by Fredie's wife, Jeannette, her son and his family. Placing the box with the groceries on the small wooden kitchen table, she peeked into the box and smiled. 'Oh, you have brought some of Fredie's favourites! He will be so happy.'

Jeanette was eighty-six years old, but despite the big age difference between them, Fredie and she had been happily married for over half a century already. 'He can still walk without support, albeit not as fast as he used to, and he still dresses himself,' she proudly told us. 'You know, he used to be a very good dancer, and that is actually how we met; at a dance. His health is still quite good, but sometimes he gets high blood pressure,' Jeanette shared. 'But he doesn't like going to the doctor. He doesn't like it when they prick his finger to take some blood, and he also doesn't like it when they put the tight armband around his arm to check his blood pressure. So, he doesn't go there much.'

She took us into the small living room and opened some of the curtains to let more light in. 'I apologize, there is no electricity at the moment, so it is a little dark here. Let me get Fredie for you.'

Fredie was born in 1904, but he didn't look his age. Nobody would guess that the man that slowly walked into the room had seen two World Wars in his lifetime and was already in his forties when apartheid was introduced in South Africa. 'I don't walk as fast as I used to,' Fredie said in Afrikaans, 'but otherwise I am okay.' He smiled, which revealed that he still had all his teeth as well. He sat down in his chair and we sat next to him and started chatting.

After telling him and his wife about what I do, I offered to teach the couple some simple yogic techniques to calm the mind and also his blood pressure, as it may be useful for him. They had never heard of yoga and meditation but were curious to find out more. After teaching them a simple breathing technique, I guided them through a short meditation. Fredie went into a very deep state of relaxation – for a moment we even thought that he had fallen asleep! After repeating the instruction to slowly open his eyes again a few more times, he finally did so. Both their kind faces now looked even brighter.

'My heart and body feel strong,' Fredie said when asked about his experience, 'and my mind feels clear and calm! I like it.' Jeanette nodded her head in agreement. 'We will practice this every day, it will be good for him, and his blood pressure.' And then she added: 'Please let us know when you can come again. I would like to invite some more people so they can learn about what you are teaching.' It was touching to see that even at this age, Fredie and his wife were so enthusiastic and open to learn and explore new things.

It is experiences like this that time and again show me that meditation is truly something that is both useful and accessible for everyone. If a gentleman like Fredie can learn to meditate, and that too at his age, why can't you? If with the right guidance he could have an authentic experience of meditation in just the first session, why wouldn't others? So, knowing that meditation is truly for everyone, let us start on this fascinating journey knowing that it is well within our reach. In the preceding chapters, we have already laid the foundation for our new meditation practice and we have learned and practised some of the important principles that will allow us to prepare the mind to relax, let go and recharge itself by moving inward.

The first thing to do is to prepare your body for meditation. Don't worry, this does not require any severe austerities or extreme flexibility, nor does it require perfect health. It does, however, require taking care of certain factors that could make it difficult to sit still and allow you to meditate properly. When the body is not comfortable, the mind will not settle down either, so we first need to make sure the body is comfortable.

Ideally, your stomach should be light and you should have finished digesting your last big meal. After a meal, your metabolism and the activity in the body goes up and all the energy goes towards your stomach, to aid in the digestive process. In meditation, however, your body goes into a state of deep rest, and your metabolism goes down. Knowing just these basics is sufficient to understand that in some ways both processes are directly opposite, and therefore both don't go together well. I am not saying that people cannot meditate properly after a meal – some may be able to sometimes. But here we are trying to make it as easy and accessible as possible for everyone, so let us go down the easy path. Just because some people have no problem jumping fences and climbing walls, it doesn't mean that all will be able to do so comfortably. So, for the average person that is already struggling to manage life's challenges and still smile, we want to make our first few strides on the path of meditation as simple and effective as possible!

With a light stomach, find a place where you will not be

disturbed much, if possible. Again, experienced meditators can happily meditate in almost any environment, so this is not a must, but a peaceful, quiet, clean and pleasant space is definitely conducive, and it will also make it much easier initially for the mind to settle down and for the body to relax.

It is not required for you to sit in a lotus posture, or even cross-legged, in order to meditate, but it does make a difference if your back is straight. It will be more comfortable in the long run, much better for your posture and it will keep your mind more alert, while relaxed, as well. It will also allow you to breathe much more comfortably, easily and deeply. Sitting in a very lazy, slouching type of posture will not be comfortable in the long run, because it will put unnecessary pressure on your neck and other parts of the body, and it also increases chances of actually dozing off when going into a more meditative state of mind. We also don't meditate lying down normally – that posture is more suitable for practices like yoga nidra, that are nowadays often referred to as 'body scan' techniques. These can also be very relaxing, but in our practice, we want to go one step further and actually meditate.

Find a position that your body is comfortable in, while sitting with your spine erect. If needed you can take back support, or sit in a comfortable chair, or sofa, if that works better for you. If you prefer sitting on the floor, but it is difficult to keep the back straight for a longer time without extra effort, then you can place a cushion or something firm below your buttocks so that you elevate your hips a little – this will make it easier to keep your back straight and take the unnecessary pressure off your lower back.

You can either cross your legs, place them on the floor or stretch them out in front of you – whatever works best for you. Just make sure that you can comfortably sit in the posture for 15-20 minutes, without having to change your position or move your legs because your legs or back were getting sore or uncomfortable.

One more thing that will really help your body, and thus also your mind, to be more comfortable during the meditation is to make sure that the body is neither very stiff, nor very restless. Especially with the sedentary lifestyle that most of us are living in today's world, where we are most of the day either sitting in the car, in the office, at home, or somewhere else, it is important to make sure to do at least a little exercise to improve the circulation and also remove any stiffness or excess energy and restlessness from the body. If you meditate in the morning before breakfast, this is important because the body will be stiff from lying in bed all night, and if you meditate in the evening after sitting in the office all day, again the body will be stiff from sitting in one posture most of the time. How you get rid of the stiffness or restlessness in the body is up to you; you can choose any way that appeals to you. Some may want to go for a run, do some yoga, put on some music and dance, or just jump up and down for a few minutes, loosening up the body and spend some energy. If you regularly find that your body is either too restless when you sit for meditation, and it is difficult to keep the body still, or you keep having a lot of restless thoughts, desires, or some sensations in the body that won't allow you to sit peacefully, then increase this exercise a little more before you sit. You can also keep an eye on your diet a little, reducing the amount of spicy, oily and fried foods you eat, and also reducing your intake of sugar.

This is actually the reason why many practitioners of yoga and meditation often end up making some changes in their food habits and diet over time – it is not that you need to follow a vegetarian or healthier diet to benefit from these practices, but the more you start becoming aware of how your body and mind react to certain types of food, and how the food you eat affects how your body and mind feel and function, you naturally start preferring things that make you feel peaceful and fresh, rather than heavy, dull, uneasy or restless.

Now that you are comfortable, having found a posture in which you can easily relax and sit still for some time, you may close your eyes and take a few slow and gentle deep breaths in and out. Take your attention to different parts of the body and consciously relax them. Here special attention can be given to the shoulders, neck and facial muscles, as these are often the places where we are most tense, and where a lot of the stress accumulates. I often tell people to keep a smile on their face – not a big grin, but just a gentle smile, as it is not possible to frown or keep a tense expression on your face and smile at the same time. So, this helps one to relax the face as well.

It is most comfortable to keep your hands on your

knees, or in your lap, with the palms open facing the sky. You don't need to keep your hands in any special postures or *mudra*, rather I would suggest not to as it again involves effort, and it does not allow you to fully relax. We often see statues of the Buddha and yogis sitting in a meditative posture while their hands form different mudras, but even though these mudras have a certain effect on our body and mind, they are also used to symbolically convey certain principles and states of mind. For us, who are starting our journey of meditation, it is important to first build a solid foundation for our practice – and that is to learn to totally relax and let go, to learn effortlessness. Keeping your hands in any specific posture will neither let your body nor your mind, relax fully. So again, let us take the easy road, and choose effortlessness over effort.

Once the body has settled into a comfortable and steady posture, take your attention to your breath for a moment. Just observe the breath, and allow it to become steady, smooth and a little slower. If you find that the breath is still a little fast, shallow or shaky, you can consciously take a few slow, long deep breaths in and out, and then again relax, allowing the breath to move at its own pace. Let the breathing be effortless as well, allowing the breath to move in and out of the body on its own. Sometimes it may be longer and deeper, and smoother and lighter, and sometimes it may be a little faster or heavier. Without putting a lot of effort to change it, just become aware of it and observe it. Become aware of how every inhalation is energizing the body, and every exhalation is relaxing the body. This is a natural phenomenon that is happening all the time, but when you begin to notice this, it becomes more effective as you are putting your attention there. And as the breath is always in the present moment, the mind also slows down, getting drawn less into the past and the future, and becoming more rooted in the present moment.

Now take your attention to any sounds or noises in the surroundings, whatever they may be. There may be the noise of the air-conditioning or a fan, there may be the noise of some people talking in another room or nearby somewhere, there may be the sounds of traffic in the distance, or some birds chirping. Whatever noises may be there, just acknowledge and accept them, allowing them to be there. Do not resist them. This is actually a technique, it is a secret, that can free your mind from those disturbances. By consciously taking your attention there and accepting the noises, you will find that the sounds become relegated to the background and they stop disturbing you. The mind then no longer gets stuck there. Otherwise, sometimes some noises can keep distracting the mind, and do not allow it to settle down. If you resist the noises, then you are stuck with the noises and the mind will not be able to go inward.

Once the mind is no longer caught up with its environment, for some time keep the body totally still. This is another secret. When the body is still, the mind also starts to further settle down, automatically, because the body and the mind are connected. When you keep the body totally still – except of course for the gentle and effortless movement of the breath – the mind also slows down more and more, even if it was active till now. So, we keep the body totally still, sitting there as if you are a statue.

Remember that the law of the mind is effortlessness, not effort. Don't put any effort to control the mind or observe it, just let it be. If it wanders, let it wander, do not resist any thoughts, while at the same time not encouraging any planning in the mind either. If there are some things that the mind is running after, some things that you still need to attend to, that you want to change, or problems that you need to solve, or things that you feel are still missing in your life, or that are not okay right now, then this is the time to practice the principle we learned in the first chapter. Consciously remind yourself that right now you don't need all those things that you thought you cannot live without. Can you be happy and peaceful without these things for now? Yes, you can be happy and peaceful even without them, in this moment.

Once this first step is done, the next is to remember the principle of dispassion. Feel that right now, this moment, you have everything you need. Right now, you don't need anything and you don't want anything. Really feel that for the next 15-20 minutes, you don't crave for anything, nor do you have to do anything. Whatever goals, desires, or items on your to-do list, they can all wait for 20 minutes.

Now consciously drop all your identities and labels. You may be a father, a mother, a lawyer, a shop attendant, a singer, a son, a sister, or anything else, but for the next 15-20 minutes drop all those identities. Feel as if you have died, as if your life has dissolved. All your relationships, all your responsibilities, all your notions and dreams. As if all of it was a dream, and you have just woken up. Feel that 'I am nothing, I am nobody.'

Unless you drop those identities, those thoughts will keep coming up. If you don't forget about your business, thoughts of pending matters, unpaid bills, tenders to be submitted, or customers to connect with, may keep coming up in your mind. But if for a moment you are able to drop all those identities, these thoughts will not even come up. So, for a moment don't give any importance to any of your identities and feel that you are nobody, that you are nothing. The past is gone, and the future is uncertain and hasn't happened yet. Dropping all your past impressions and ideas about yourself and your life so far, as well as dropping the plans for the future. During your time of meditation, you don't want to do anything. You are new this moment, in this moment. And right now, you don't have to do anything. Dropping the past completely, and not getting lost in our plans for the future either – we learned and practised this in the second chapter, remember? And we learned to drop all our identities, all our labels, and everything that is going on in our life right now, in the fourth chapter in detail.

The above application of the practice of dispassion culminates in three beautiful principles that I have learned from my Master. He taught us these as a preparation for meditation. Summed up, the three principles are feeling that for the next few moments:

(1) I am nothing,
(2) I want nothing, and
(3) I don't have to do anything.

For a moment consciously bringing these to your awareness and really feeling it is a technique that can really allow you to go into meditation much faster. Feel that right now, for the next few moments, you are nothing, you are nobody, and you want nothing, and right now, you don't have to do anything. And when you can feel this, you will find that the mind starts settling down. Many of the usual thoughts will not even come up now.

This is the point where you relax and let go. If some thoughts come up, just let them come and go on their own. We don't label or entertain them. Thoughts come and go on their own, we don't analyse them. Whether good thoughts or bad thoughts, do not resist, just let them be there. They come and go, like waves rising from the ocean, only to dissolve back into it. Just like waves, these thoughts are just there on the surface of your consciousness. The more they settle, the stiller the surface becomes, and the more you are able to see and appreciate the depth of the ocean of your consciousness.

If you find, however, that your mind is stuck with a thought, that it keeps coming back, or if you notice that some planning is going on in the mind, gently bring it back to the present moment by momentarily taking your attention to your breath. We have practised this already in the fifth chapter as well, remember?

Accept whatever is happening and embrace it. If there are a lot of thoughts, let it be, it is okay. Don't try to quickly get rid of it or quickly relax – it doesn't work. The more you are able to accept and just be with whatever is happening, the more both body and mind will settle down and become peaceful. Meditation is de-concentration; it is the art of letting go and just being. The more you are able to 'let go', the more you will be able to go deep in meditation. And this includes even letting go of the desire to 'meditate well' or 'to go deep in meditation'.

I have experienced at different times when sitting for meditation that something was disturbing me or that my mind kept thinking about something, and that it made it impossible for me to go deep in meditation. However, the moment that I decided that even if meditation doesn't happen, I am okay with it, and that I will just sit for those 15-20 minutes, no matter what happens, the meditation suddenly started becoming deeper. Giving up the desire to meditate, and dropping the 'doership', are an essential and very powerful step in the process of meditation. Here the fastest way to reach the goal is to have infinite patience!

There is a beautiful story that is sometimes used to illustrate this point of the meditation practice or any other spiritual practices. There are different versions of this story that I have come across over the years, but the way I heard it for the first time many years ago goes something like this.

One day a Master decided to go for a walk around his Ashram, and seeing the disciples involved in their service activities and spiritual practices, he smiled to himself. He was getting old and he knew that his body had only a few years left to live.

At this moment, one of his most senior disciples who was accompanying him, turned to the Master and with a serious look on his face asked, 'Master, I have been with you with for the last few decades, and I have been sincere in my meditation practice. However, you yourself have told us that you will be with us in this body for only a few more years. Please tell me, when will I reach enlightenment? When will I be liberated?'

Seeing the longing in the eyes of the disciple, the Master closed his eyes for a moment and used his divine intuition. Opening his eyes again, he looked at the disciple with a lot of compassion, and told him: 'It will take you four more lifetimes to reach enlightenment and become liberated my son.'

Hearing this, the senior disciple's face turned grey, and then this made way for anger. 'What? Four lifetimes? But I have given most of my life to you and your teachings. I have been doing my practices sincerely for the last few decades! This is outrageous.'

Having overheard the conversation between the senior disciple and the Master, a young boy, who had joined the Ashram only a few years ago, hesitatingly approached the Master, and in all his innocence asked: 'Master, what about me? Could you tell me when I will be liberated?'

Once more the Master closed his eyes for a moment, and when he opened his eyes again, he smiled at the boy and told him: 'Do you see that tree over there that you were watering? And do you see all the leaves on the branches of the tree?'

'Yes Master,' the boy replied happily, 'I see them!'

'Well, my boy, it will take you as many lifetimes as there are leaves on that tree before you attain enlightenment.' The boy's smile became even bigger, and gratefully he bowed down to the Master.

The senior disciple, who was still angry, turned to the boy and asked him: 'Why are you so happy? Don't you see there are thousands of leaves on that tree?'

'Oh yes, I see them. But I am so happy because I can count the number of leaves on this tree, it is a finite number. There may be thousands, yes, but the Master has just told me that I will get enlightened, once these are over.'

Tears of joy and gratitude rolling down his cheeks, the young boy started dancing in joy, feeling so happy that he would get enlightened one day. And it is said that at that moment enlightenment dawned on the boy and he became liberated.

One of the beautiful lessons that this story carries is that the fastest way to reach the goal in meditation or any spiritual practices is to not be in a hurry but to have infinite patience. This of course does not mean that you just sit there waiting or keep on doing other things; it means that you are able to practice without the feverishness of wanting to achieve a certain goal or experience. Having infinite patience means having the ability to practice without any restlessness or craving for any experiences or results in the mind. Applying yourself fully to the action, while dropping the desire for the fruit of the action, or the outcome. It will allow you to be fully in the present moment and truly go deep, as the mind is able to fully relax. Wanting something to happen is still doing something – and as we saw earlier, meditation is the art of doing nothing, the art of letting go. So, here we also apply the principle that we learned in chapter three: the ability to just be with what we are doing, completely, forgetting about all the times you have already done this in the past, and how our experiences were then. Sitting as if you are meditating for the first time, knowing that every time you sit for meditation it is a new experience, and forgetting everything you think you know about it, and what is supposed to happen. Dropping all the earlier experiences, be it good or bad, and just being fully available to experience whatever is happening right now. Forget about what you are supposed to gain from it, or how it will benefit you, and just practice with childlike innocence and enthusiasm, without worrying about the result.

The more you are able to practice dispassion like this, the more you will be able to drop even the desire to meditate or be peaceful. And the more this happens, the more effortless, deep and profound your meditations become, and the more joyful, peaceful and free you will be.

The first sign is that after your meditation you feel more relaxed, fresher, more centred and the mind is calmer. In some meditations, you may not have felt the time pass, or you may not have been aware of much at all, while at other times you may have an acute awareness and yet the mind is very relaxed. You may have initially felt that you had so many thoughts, as you were aware of them, but then seeing that twenty minutes have already passed, it may suddenly strike you that you did not have *those* many thoughts. This means that there were gaps of thoughtlessness in between, where you were not even aware at all – you had transcended the logical mind. But despite the feeling that you had many thoughts, you feel rested afterwards.

Every time you sit for meditation the experiences may differ, so it is very important not to judge yourself or your experiences in meditation or try to analyse them too much. It is also important not to compare your experiences too much with others, or with things that you have read or heard about. There are so many funny concepts and misconceptions about meditation floating around, and many people get stuck with those ideas. I have had people coming to me to get guidance in their meditation practice, saying they have still not been able to see the bright light that they had read about somewhere and that was supposedly the indication of meditation happening. The poor souls had been desperately trying to see a bright light, which had only made their attempts more stressful and tiring for the mind, rather than them actually feeling better and more peaceful. All kinds of experiences can come in meditation, but we don't get stuck with them or get attached to them. If you practice regularly, you may see some colours, smell some fragrance, have some sensations as if you are floating, or you may feel very light, or heavy, and all kinds of other experiences – or you may have none of these at all.

Looking for such experiences or trying to recreate them is one more place where people sometimes get stuck. As my Master once beautifully said when someone asked him about some of these experiences that one of their friends had gone through, but they hadn't: 'Meditation is not about the experience, it is about the experiencer.' So, don't get stuck with experiences, comparing your own with others or judging yourself. Take every time you sit for meditation as a new experience, and welcome whatever comes with open arms. This innocence and state of surrender is another very important aspect and powerful tool to go deep in one's meditation practice. Because like I shared earlier, meditation is an art or skill that comes by practice, not by knowing something intellectually. I have of course shared certain guidelines, principles and tips with you, but more important than that is having an innocent mind that is willing to embrace and experience the unknown. Because meditation is going beyond the mind, and therefore, it can never be known intellectually, only experienced.

There is a beautiful short story that illustrates this childlike innocence and the importance of our approach and state of mind over the technical know-how of the technique. This story was written by Leo Tolstoy at the end of the nineteenth century, but its message is as true today as it was then.

The story tells us about three hermits that lived on a small island somewhere in a big lake in a remote part of Russia. Over time word spread about the three saints and the miracles they performed, and the local bishop became worried that the popularity of these hermits may start affecting the position and authority of the church in these regions. After contemplating the problem, the bishop came up with a solution: he would visit the old men and teach them the ways of the church. This way, even if people still considered them as saints, it would not lead them away from the churchly traditions.

The next day the bishop set out for the lake and upon reaching the shore, he requested the captain of a fisherman's boat to take him to the remote island where the three men were living. When asked if he knew about the three saints, the captain replied that he had heard stories from the local people about some of the miracles that the saints perform. 'But I don't think going there is worth your time, your eminence,' the captain added. 'From what I have heard, these saints are simple people and not very educated.'

The bishop, however, was adamant about wanting to visit these hermits, and the captain agreed to take him to the island. Having come near, he provided the bishop with a small rowboat as the main ship could not go further in the shallow waters near the island. The captain promised to wait for the bishop to return.

Having reached the shore, the bishop was received by the three saints, who appeared to just look like three old poor men, living a very simple life of austerities there.

'I have heard about your earnest quest for God and salvation,' the bishop told them, 'and I find your dedication quite admirable. Could you tell me how you are seeking God and His mercy? How do you pray?'

The three saints looked at each other for a moment, and then one of them reluctantly told the bishop that they actually did not really know how to pray or serve God. Their prayer, in all its innocence, was simple: 'Three are ye, three are we, have mercy upon us.'

Having heard this, the bishop explained to them that even though their intention was pure, their prayer was not proper. He then went on to teach them how one was supposed to pray as per the holy scriptures that God had given to men. He explained to them the various doctrines that have been mentioned in the holy scriptures, and then taught them the Lord's Prayer, known as the 'Our Father'.

This turned out to be a big challenge though, as the men had great difficulty in remembering the correct words of the prayer. By the time the bishop was confident that the hermits had finally memorized the prayer, it had already become nighttime. Once more emphasizing to the three men the need to pray only in this correct manner, the bishop then got back to his rowboat and returned to the fisherman's ship.

The bishop boarded the ship, but then as the captain turned the boat and started sailing back towards the shore of the big lake, a small light appeared in the dark behind them. Initially, the bishop thought it must be another small boat that was also on its way to the shore, but as the faint light drew closer, he suddenly saw that the small lamp was held up by one of the three hermits as all three of them came running towards the boat.

The bishop, in all his astonishment of seeing these men run on water as if they were on solid ground, quickly asked the captain to stop the boat. As the saints reached the boat, they humbly greeted the bishop, and after catching their breath for a moment, one of them asked him, 'Your eminence, please forgive us, but we have forgotten your teachings again. As long as we kept repeating the prayer you taught us, we were able to remember it. But when we took a small break, we realized we had forgotten some of the words, and before we knew it, we could not remember any of them properly anymore. Please teach it to us once more!'

Realizing that the old men were truly saints, having been blessed by God, the humbled bishop realized his mistake. 'My dear brothers, it was my ignorance to think that I can teach you anything about faith and how to serve our heavenly Father. Please continue praying in your own way, as you have done till now. Your prayers reach the Lord, there is no doubt about that. Please pray for all of us sinners.' Feeling relieved, the three saints happily returned to their small island, walking across the surface of the lake.

This story touches upon another important aspect of an authentic meditation practice as well, and that is having a sense of honour and respect, or reverence for the practice. I feel it is important to explore this a little more in detail here, because with the commercialization and so-called secularization of meditation over the last few decades, some important aspects of this ancient practice have knowingly or unknowingly taken a backseat or have even been removed altogether.

We currently live in a time where meditation has become so fashionable and lucrative, that there are not just a few but many meditation apps for your phone, iPads and other devices, and many offer premium subscription packages that allow you to unlock an even wider range of quick-fix meditations. You have options that cater to all types of hectic lifestyles, with some apps even offering 'meditations' as short as one or two minutes – short enough to fit into the tightest of schedules, with the promise of giving you more peace of mind or space in your head. Most of these meditations have been 'invented' or developed by people that may have very limited or no knowledge or understanding of the ancient traditions and context in which these powerful practices were taught and practised, and this results in many of the so-called 'meditations' being actually more like snippets of soothing nature sounds or instrumental music with a picture of some beautiful landscape in the background, or worse.

It seems that in an effort to make the concept and practice of meditation more accessible and less foreign for the masses, many have tried to remove the cultural or spiritual elements and context of the practice, in a similar way as yoga has in many places undergone such a transformation – or sometimes I would even say distortion. One of the reasons that the word 'mindfulness' and 'meditation' are frequently used interchangeably is that still many corporates and other institutions seem to be a little hesitant, to say the least, in introducing anything culturally or religiously coloured as meditation to their executives and employees, while something as secular and neutral as mindfulness is much less of an 'issue'. The world has come a long way, and we are much more open-minded than a few centuries ago, but it is in instances like these that one realizes that still not all embrace wisdom and useful techniques from all over the world, in the same way, they have happily embraced clothes, fashion, technology, food, music and movies from across the globe.

We shouldn't shy away from the traditions that meditation came from though, as in an over-zealous effort to secularize things, we often end up throwing away the baby with the bathwater, where we strip the practice of some of the elements that actually form its very essence. Of course, one does not have to be a Buddhist, or a Hindu, or a follower of any other religion for that matter, in order to be able to practice meditation and benefit from it. But a sense of honour, reverence and respect for the practice and the tradition, and a sense of faith in oneself, the technique and the teacher are very important aspects of the meditation practice, or any spiritual practice for that matter. Because if you look at honouring, at having a sense of reverence, then you will see that it is nothing but a total attentiveness of the mind, coupled with a tinge of gratitude.

Whether it is you receiving a guest at home or picking up a book or object that you have a lot of reverence for, in both instances, you will find that your mind comes fully to the present moment, coupled with a subtle feeling of gratefulness and happiness. A random person walking into your home does not invoke a similar state of your mind or consciousness, nor does picking up an old newspaper and putting it away somewhere else. And this is exactly why in ancient times so much emphasis was given to honouring the Master, the practice and the tradition.

The whole purpose of meditation is to consolidate the mind, to bring it back to a calm and composed state from its scattered and chaotic condition and to allow it to settle down and finally transcend itself. The moment one sits down with a sense of reverence for the practice, more than half the job is already done. But if this aspect is missing, the meditation practice many times takes on the form of mere mental exercise, where one desperately tries to calm a restless mind. And then people wonder why it is so difficult to even just focus the mind on any one thing for more than a few seconds. Those who have joined some mindfulness classes may have realized that really being mindful or aware turns out to be much more easily said than done. You would think that just the awareness of the need to be in the present moment with what you are doing right now would allow one to consciously practice it – why would you need a course or training? But the truth is that many are not able to do this so easily and becoming conscious of this fact often only adds to the tension, leaving a beginner more disheartened than hopeful of achieving that coveted state of inner peace.

The monks, meditation masters and the icons of liberation and enlightenment, like the great saints and sages of the ancient yogic traditions, including the Buddha, all share the common ground of a practice that is rooted in and part of an ancient tradition that has perfected it and that has preserved it and handed it down through a system of masters and disciples, and a reverence for the tradition.

But when meditation became interesting from a big business point of view, the over-enthusiastic marketing departments lost no time in stripping it of many of its cultural and traditional baggage, in an attempt to make it as modern as the gym around the corner. Peace of mind at your fingertips, and that too at very affordable rates. One of the leading apps proudly boasts to offer 3-minute sessions that fit seamlessly into a busy schedule – just the thought itself can actually make you more stressed! Honestly, anyone who has any authentic experience of true meditation can tell you that this has become something very different, no matter how big an expert someone may claim to be. It is therefore also not very surprising that most studies of the modern mindfulness apps available for your phones and tablets show that there is hardly any evidence at all of these apps actually working, or even remotely doing what they promise their users they will do. The people making these apps may have the knowledge of branding, coding and designing, but they may not be masters of a tradition that has perfected and preserved these ancient techniques with sacredness and proper understanding.

I have come across so many people who have started referring to their meditation workshops or practices as mindfulness, because they feel it appeals much more to the mainstream crowd and I have even heard people refer to the arrival of 'secular mindfulness' that made it even more accessible for people from all backgrounds and walks of life. I often feel that this obsession with wanting everything to be secular and stripped of anything that could be interpreted as even vaguely religious has done more damage than good. Has religion as such gotten such a bad name in today's world that anything vaguely or potentially religious is synonymous with blind belief, a distorted view of reality and dogmas? Or is there this underlying fear that you may accidentally end up practising something that is part of some other religion than your own? Is our faith really that shaky – be it in our own rational mind and thinking, or in our own religion, if we follow any?

Of course, we also see the other extreme, where some may make you feel like the only way to meditate properly is to leave all that you know behind and join a retreat in a mountain spa or a monastery far away from civilization. Again, the truth does not lie in the extremes, but in the middle path. Nobody will argue that a peaceful retreat in the stillness of nature, with the soothing view of mountain ranges or the ocean will help you settle down and be less distracted, but that does not mean that you cannot learn to meditate and experience true stillness in the comfort of your home. Rather, a practice that is compatible with your existing day-to-day life and routine stands a much better chance of truly helping you to become more peaceful and resilient in the long run.

The reason why I wanted to address these points is because I have seen more often than not that by taking these ancient, time-tested and beneficial practices and techniques out of their context, tradition and culture often results in stripping it of some of its essential aspects as well. The ancient Vedic and Yogic traditions have always welcomed a scientific and inquisitive approach, rather they encourage it. It is the foundation of these systems of philosophy and practices, and that is how thousands of years ago the sages with their scientific mindset went on to explore and develop these ancient techniques, like meditation. They knew, however, that in order to learn and be open to experience something, a receptive mindset and reverence for the teachings and practice are of great importance, as we are dealing here with something as subtle as our mind. So, bringing in this element of respect and reverence for the practice can really help you, and make it much easier to manage your mind and learn how to actually meditate.

During the early years of my martial arts practice, I noticed how even in our training the reverence and respect for the master and the tradition played an important role, and how that in turn actually made it much easier to learn new things. Because the reverence and respect were there, the mind was naturally more focused, more aware, and more in the present moment. And when I met Gurudev Sri Sri Ravi Shankar and experienced what it was like to meditate with him, under his guidance, I realized that I had finally found a true meditation master.

I have been learning from him for the last twenty years and have also learned many things from him personally. The power of tradition, of tried and tested techniques offered and explained by someone who has truly mastered them, is a completely different experience than trying to figure something out on your own. Thus, adding this element of reverence for the technique and the practice will really help you.

And that is how you will keep going deeper into the practice, and it will give you so many benefits. The more you learn to relax the mind and for a moment allow it to turn inward and settle down, the more the mind starts expanding. A mind that is tense feels as if it contracts, and the more you relax, the more there is a feeling of expansion. And the more the body and mind settle down and go into a state of rest, the more your system will start releasing built up stresses and strains.

You are allowing the nervous system and mind to rejuvenate itself, and in the process, they unburden themselves from unwanted impressions and strains. You may therefore experience these releases happening on three different levels: in the physical, mental or emotional sphere. On the physical level you may feel some stiffness, discomfort or some tingling sensations. You may even have a sudden jerk of one of your arms or so, if a muscle was very tight and it suddenly relaxes.

When I started meditating regularly, I remember wondering why as soon as five minutes into my meditation I would sometimes start feeling some pain in my back, or some stiffness in my legs, while I had no problem sitting in the same position while watching TV or a movie, even if it was for more than an hour. First, I thought that maybe it is just because while watching TV, I am not as conscious or aware of my body and how it feels, but I learned that it is not just that. In meditation the body is able to throw of so many pent-up stresses and strains, and one of the ways this gets released is on the physical level.

You may also sometimes find that while meditating you start getting a lot of thoughts, effortlessly, about all kinds of random things. You are not consciously thinking or remembering things, nor are you actively planning something in your mind. These are just random thoughts, coming in one after another, and these may just be impressions that are getting released because the mind is finally settling down. So, this does not mean that your meditation is not happening, or that it is not working – you are doing it right, and that is why this release occurs. You will find that with regular practice these thoughts will become fewer, as you have started clearing out all the backlog of unnecessary impressions that have been putting a strain on your nervous system. If thoughts come, it's not a problem. Let them. Whether good or bad, positive or negative, let them. Don't label them, because then you will want to hold on to or entertain the good thoughts and resist the bad ones. The art of doing nothing means . . . doing nothing. So, also when a thought comes, we do nothing. And just like a car that was driving very fast takes some time to come to a standstill, even if you apply the brakes fully, the mind will initially also be active sometimes, but we just let it settle down, give it time. We are dropping the effort, the concentration, the observing and letting go, just being. The initial focus or awareness of the surroundings, of our body, of our breath, is not the goal – they are a means to bring together and consolidate the scattered mind before it can drop even that.

It is like how the scriptures also describe one of the ways to liberation or freedom: have one desire, to be free, that is so intense, that it makes you drop all others, and when only that remains, drop that also. Like that one strong desire that dissolves all others, the initial awareness of the mind is like the alum that is put in the water to purify it, and that then dissolves itself, leaving nothing but pure water. Here we see that most of the commonly practised mindfulness practices and meditations are actually just the preparation part, not the actual meditation. They never go beyond the mind.

Finally, it is also possible for different emotions to come up during meditation. Here it is again important to remember that if and when this happens, we don't need to analyse them because these are just releases happening to unburden your system. We hardly ever stop to think about the impact that not expressing our emotions has on us. Of course, we often cannot, and should not, express it when we feel angry or annoyed or frustrated, because we live in a society and we follow certain rules of decency. Imagine if you did not hold back and fully expressed your anger every time your annoying boss took credit for your work? You will lose your job in no time! In the same way, you cannot always express your displeasure with a certain member of your family every time you feel that way because your home will soon turn into a warzone. But not expressing an emotion does not mean we don't feel it, and every time we go through it, it leaves some impact on our nervous system, even on a hormonal level. And when we allow our body and mind to rest deeply, they naturally start releasing these unnecessary burdens on the system.

The more you become rested and peaceful, free from stresses, strains and worries, you will find that all those things that you have been looking for and running after, like happiness, peace, a sense of freedom and well-being, are already there. It was just covered with all the mental clouds and now the sun of your true nature can shine through again. Just like when you were a small child. So now all that is left is to find the time to make meditation a part of your life.

Wisdom Sutras

- Meditation is a skill that comes by practice, not by knowing something intellectually.
- Reverence greatly enhances your meditation practice. It is a state of mind where the mind is fully focused, in the present moment, with a sense of joy and gratitude, effortlessly.

10-Minute Exercise

Practice the process that has been described in this chapter to start meditating. Familiarize yourself with the main steps, and then just let go and enjoy the practice. Remember the story of the three innocent saints: your feeling and sincerity is more important than following all instructions by the letter. As a general rule you could keep the following principles in mind, as they will be useful, whether you are new to meditation, or have been meditating already:

1. Find a proper place to sit without much disturbance, and prepare your body by having a light stomach, and doing a little exercise or stretches to warm up and loosen up the body.
2. Sit in a comfortable posture with your spine erect, and then consciously relax the entire body. Become aware of any noises around you and accept them, let them be.
3. Allow the breath to settle down, and then keep the body still. Allow the mind to settle down even more.

4. Drop all your pending work, desires, ambitions, identities and labels. For the next few moments, you are totally content in this present moment. You are nothing, want nothing, and don't have to do anything right now.
5. Now totally relax, allowing thoughts and sensations in the body to come and go on their own, as and when they come.
6. When you are done, take one to two minutes to gradually come out of the meditation, before you open your eyes and go back to your other activities.

It is always recommended to learn any meditation technique from an actual teacher, at least initially, so that they can guide you personally. But for those who are still new to meditation, and are yet to explore the beautiful programs we offer, a great place to start maybe some of the guided meditations of my Master, Gurudev Sri Sri Ravi Shankar. He also regularly conducts meditations online via his YouTube channel. Meditating in the presence of a realised Master is a profound experience, and so much more effortless. It is worth experiencing!

7

Finding the Time to Meditate

Like many train stations in Assam, Diphu station is not very big, and my train would only stop there for a few minutes. Seeing many of the coaches rushing by already, the long train came to a screeching halt. 'Swamiji, your coach has already passed. We will have to go to the end of the platform! I will take this bag.'

One of the volunteers that had come to drop me off at the station took my suitcase and carrying my backpack myself, we quickly ran to the end of the platform, dodging people that were getting off the train as well as those trying to get on it in time, while also being careful not to step on some of the people whose train had been delayed, and who had decided to get comfortable and were sitting or lying down on the same platform.

We found the carriage and quickly went inside. 'Swamiji, this is your place. Seat number 12, lower berth. Excuse us,

Sir.' The volunteer placed my bag under the seat after the gentleman already sitting there moved aside a little. 'Are you comfortable here? Do you need anything else? We hope you will come back again to Karbi Anglong!'

'I hope so too!' I replied to the volunteer and thanked him for his help. 'Don't worry, I am comfortable. You go, the train is about to start moving.' Quickly touching my feet in a gesture of respect, the boy ran off, jumping onto the platform just in time as the train was now slowly rolling out of the station.

Placing my small backpack next to me on the seat, I placed my shoes below the seat, pulled up my legs and sat back a little. The benefit of travelling by sleeper class is that the beds allow for one to sit comfortably in a cross-legged position as well. I checked the time on my phone and realized there was about half an hour left before they would start serving the dinner parcels on the train – this gave me just enough time without any disturbance. I closed my eyes, relaxed my shoulders, took a few long deep breaths, allowed the breathing to settle and started my evening meditation. Soon the sounds of the train rolling over the railway tracks, the children talking in the compartment next to me, and a person listening to music on his mobile phone started fading into the background until they no longer caught my attention. For a moment I became aware of the sound of the air-conditioning in the coach trying to keep up with the hot and humid air that had come into the carriage with us from the outside – weather that was typical for this time of the year in these parts of Assam – and then even that disappeared from my awareness. The mind started expanding, and before I knew it what remained was just a subtle awareness of the body moving back and forth, or left and right a little, swaying along with the carriage of the train as it moved across the not entirely even tracks or terrain. The body and mind had gone into a deep state of relaxation, and all that remained was a sense of gradual expansion. When I finally became more aware of the body and mind again, I took a few moments to become aware of my surroundings as well, before I opened my eyes again. About 25 minutes had passed, and I felt much fresher. My mind was also much more settled.

Opening my eyes, I looked at the smiling and curious face of the gentleman that had been sitting in my place when we had boarded the train. It appeared his seat was opposite of me. 'Were you meditating?' He asked me hesitantly. 'I hope you don't mind me asking.'

'I don't mind at all,' I replied, 'And yes, I was.'

'I noticed your dress, and the way the boy who accompanied you interacted with you. Are you working for some spiritual organization? Hare Krishna? You speak Hindi fluently, but you look like you have come from abroad?'

I smiled. 'Yes, I am originally from the Netherlands, but I have been living in India for the last ten years now. I am a disciple of Gurudev Sri Sri Ravi Shankar, the founder of The Art of Living. You must have heard of him?'

'Oh yes, yes, I have seen some of his discourses on TV. I like him, he speaks in very easy language, it is not difficult to understand. So, you came here for work?'

'Yes, I am overseeing many of our humanitarian service projects of the organization in the North Eastern Region, and I just finished conducting a meditation retreat and some yoga programs here in Diphu.'

'Oh yes, I saw you were meditating. I also tried it for some time, but I can't get my mind to stop thinking. I go for a morning walk every day though. Well, not every day, but as often as I can. You know how it is, nowadays we have much less time for these things.'

What this man told me was right. One of the biggest challenges in life is finding the time to do the things that are really important for us, or that you know you should be doing. This is one of the main things that distinguishes successful people from the rest – and here successful does not only refer to those with a high-level position in their company or those with a big bank balance. Here I am mainly talking about the people who are truly happy, contented, fulfilled, grateful and peaceful in life, no matter what their profession, social status or income is like.

It is not that most of us don't know what is important, or what is important to us, but we keep saying that we don't get time to do those things, not realizing that in order to get time, you have to make time. If you keep waiting for the day that you will finally get time to do those things you have been postponing, it will most probably never happen. Unless, of course, there is a sudden pandemic and life suddenly comes to a standstill. Apart from all the negative impact that the lockdown has had on people across the world, it has also resulted in almost everybody I know finally getting some time and space to do things that they had been wanting to do for a very long time, even years, but they were simply not getting time for. And in the process, it also led to many people re-evaluating their lives, and where they were heading, and what they want to do with their lives. In this way, I know that for many this sudden interruption of their busy lifestyles has also been a blessing in disguise. A moment to slow down, introspect and look inward.

Let's face it, life has become much more hectic in the last few decades, and it only continues to speed up. Everything is faster, and it is becoming more and more common to 'have to schedule some time' for the most basic things in life, be it meals, exercise or some time with your family.

I remember the time of my primary school days, before we all had mobile phones and voicemail or messenger apps. If you had to call someone, you would pick up the landline phone, dial their number and if you got lucky, they answered. If they did not, you had to presume that they were either busy or unavailable, and you would just have to try again later. With mobile phones the scenario changed, as people started carrying them wherever they went, and nowadays you can even see whether someone is 'online' on most messenger apps. If you don't pick up their call, someone will message you, and if you don't reply within a few minutes, you sometimes even have to justify why you didn't reply right away. Your boss may expect a reply to the email they just forwarded to you within the hour and may not appreciate it if you don't call them back immediately after you missed their call. Nobody considers that you may be busy right now, or even worse, may actually have a life. However, in this rat-race where we try to squeeze maximum activities and experiences into the same 24 hours of our day, we often end up running after things that promise us the peace and happiness that we are looking for, while that lasting joy and fulfilment seems to keep slipping through our fingers. We manage to do two or three things at the same time, and in the process miss out on fully experiencing or enjoying any of them. There is a short parable by Leo Tolstoy that beautifully captures our predicament, and it goes something like this.

Once upon a time, there lived a man in India who had lost all that he had. Dejected and having given up on life, he sat on the side of the road just outside the town, near a local temple, begging the people passing by to give him some change. There was not a day that the beggar was not found sitting there, on that same spot, begging anyone that passed by to give him something. Many years passed and the beggar became old, until one day he finally passed away.

Kind as they were, the workers of the nearby temple decided to arrange for the final rites to be performed for the man, and so they did. And after this was done, they decided to clean up the place where the beggar had been living all these years. They removed all the rags and clutter, and also decided to dig up some of the soil of the place and take it away.

As they were cleaning the area, one of them stumbled upon something hard in the ground. Removing a little more of the earth, they discovered a heavy pot that had been buried there and upon opening the cover they saw that it was filled with gold coins. Shaking their heads at the irony, they realized that the poor man who had been asking all passers-by for small change for years had actually been sitting on such a treasure all this time, without ever finding out. Sitting on such riches, he had died a poor and miserable man.

And before we judge this beggar, we better introspect as in some ways we are not that different. Remember the story of Mullah who was looking for the keys outside of his house, while he lost them inside? We say we don't have time to meditate, to look inward, but why is that? It is because we are so busy trying to gain things, achieve things, and experience things that somehow promise us the peace, joy, fulfilment, love and sense of freedom that we are looking for. But what we have learned, and what we have realized in the earlier chapters of this book, is that it is in the end exactly that, just a promise. It is a promise of happiness later, never now. And we realized that true happiness is only in the present moment, it is only now, never later. And it can only be experienced when the mind becomes calm, when it comes to the present moment, and when we become free from the burden of the past and the uncertainty of the future.

We need to realize that the switch is inside and that we are ignoring the shortcut that has been presented to us, trying to reach our goal via a much longer route, that may or may not even lead us there.

Remember the joy, freedom and peace that we have all known as small children and know that you have not lost it forever. It is still there, inside, but it has been covered by the mud and dust of stress, desires, craving and aversion, and limitless ambition. When you remove this dirt, you will find the treasure that was buried there all along, and that has all this time been within your reach. And this is not as difficult as you may think, but it does need awareness and understanding, along with a pinch of commitment.

The awareness has already dawned, as we have discovered in the earlier chapters how relevant and important it is to make meditation a part of our life. We also saw that it requires us to actually slow down for a moment and be totally with what we are doing, rather than just downloading an app for a three- or five-minute meditation, packaged and marketed to fit in perfectly with our fast-food and multi-task culture – something that is contradictory to what meditation is all about. However, that does not mean that meditation is not for people with busy lives and a hectic schedule – rather it is the opposite. Meditation is all the more needed when we live a busy and stressful life; more than a luxury, it becomes a necessity, if you want to maintain a certain level of happiness and productivity.

But awareness of the problem and the solution alone is

not sufficient. For you to get to the point where you actually start 'doing' it, you need to also really understand why is it important. You may have read a book about delicious cakes with elaborate descriptions, beautiful pictures and all the instructions on how to make them, but unless you make some and eat them it will never give you the experience that actually eating a piece of pie does, nor will it fill your stomach. You can read all the books you want about changing your life, but nothing will happen unless you decide to do it, and that comes from acknowledging the importance you need to give it because life is all about priorities. You have read about the importance of being in the present moment, of the mind being peaceful, here and now, free from cravings and aversions, but all that is useless unless you experience it. And that is why we need to meditate – to actually experience that state of mind, to realize it. Because otherwise, it is no different from expecting your stomach to be filled just by reading the menu card – it will never happen.

I know many people who wanted to quit smoking but only very few did it. They all know that it is bad for their health and that it may even cause lung cancer in the long run, and yet this doesn't stop them from lighting another cigarette. Everybody 'knows' that it is bad for your health, but very few actually 'understand' what this really means. In the same way, I know some people who were able to quit smoking overnight when they were suddenly confronted with the death of a close friend or relative – be it due to lung cancer or a similar condition. Suddenly the dangers or suffering of such a condition became very real for them – they finally 'understood'. And when this understanding dawned, it made quitting smoking that much easier for them. It now seemed like such an obvious thing to do.

I could give many more examples of cases where people suddenly 'understood' the importance of doing something, whether it was exercising, changing their diet, following traffic rules, or anything else, and it allowed them to change their habits or priorities overnight. It is just a matter of you realizing the importance of what you are doing. After all, you always find time to eat something, albeit a little late maybe, no matter how busy your day was. Why? Because you know it is important. In the same way, you make sure that you take a bath and brush your teeth before going for an important meeting, no matter how tight your schedule is, right? Well, I sincerely hope you do, for your sake, and for the others you will be meeting.

You have made it a habit to take a bath and brush your teeth every day because at some point in life you realized that it is important. When you were small your parents had to maybe tell you, or force you, to brush your teeth, but now you don't need anyone to tell you or remind you. In the same way, we need to understand that in our modern world it is necessary to make meditation a part of our daily routine as well. As my Master puts it aptly, 'We have understood the importance of dental hygiene, but we have often neglected to take care of our mental hygiene.' So just like you take a shower to clean and refresh the body once or twice a day, we need to meditate once or twice a day to clean and refresh our mind as well. And don't worry 15-20 minutes is enough, just like when you take a shower. We don't spend hours in the shower, or brushing our teeth, and in the same way, we don't have to give up all the other things in our life just because we want to meditate. It does, however, require you to revisit your priorities a little. It does need a little bit of discipline and commitment.

And before you freak out and go into a rebel-mindset because the first thing that comes to mind when you hear the words discipline and commitment is you losing all your freedom and precious time, let us address this misconception. We often feel that a discipline or routine robs us of our freedom to do what we want when we want. It binds and restricts us. But the interesting thing is that it is actually the other way around.

If you look closely at your life, you will realize that it is the disciplines you have that make you more comfortable and freer. Your discipline of brushing your teeth saves you from toothache, bad breath and other discomforts. It makes you freer, as nobody with a toothache or half his teeth would be very comfortable. Your discipline in your diet keeps you more healthy and fit. People who have no discipline in their diet often end up being unhealthy and they end up suffering all kinds of discomforts and ailments, leaving them much less peaceful than you are. In the same way, having a discipline of exercising makes your body fitter, more comfortable and it makes you feel better overall. You may not have any of the stiffness, pains and aches and other discomforts that your colleagues experience due to many hours of sitting in the office, without taking time out to exercise the body a little.

I know people who would tell me they felt bad for me that I have to get up early every day to do some exercise, some yoga, to do my breathwork techniques and meditation, while they got to use their morning to sleep in. They did not realize that that little investment in the morning not only makes me healthier but also lets me be at ease throughout the day, and much more effective at all my tasks. Taking out that extra time for meditation ends up adding a lot more energy and efficiency to your day. Not just that, since meditation helps the mind relax, you will observe a great improvement in the quality of your sleep.

I have had people who fell asleep during their first meditation sessions with me, because their body was so tired that when it relaxed so deeply, it took the rest that it desperately needed. And that is also fine. They felt so good afterwards, and once the body and mind became more rested, they were able to meditate as well.

In the same way, people often share a drastic improvement in the quality of their sleep once they start becoming regular with their meditation practice, because the mind is much more peaceful, and it is becoming better at really 'letting go' at night as well. After all, true rest can only happen when you drop everything else that you are doing, including all your plans, worries and ambitions. Whenever you are not able to do that, your sleep isn't as peaceful. We would have all experienced at some point or other that you may even end up dreaming about those issues or plans that were still going through your head when you hit the bed. In meditation, we learn how to really drop everything, even if it is just for a while.

Once you have really 'understood' that making this discipline part of your daily routine is the most intelligent thing to do, all that is left is to just do it, and to become regular with your practice. The more regular you are with your practice, the easier and more effortless it becomes. Even in the ancient scriptures on yoga and meditation, continuity in the practice has been given an important place, as that is what will really help you make it part of your life, especially in the beginning, and it will also give you the maximum benefits of the practice. It is said that anything that is practised for forty-eight consecutive days becomes a habit, and if you continue doing it without a break long enough, becomes part of your nature. Ask any athlete or person that exercises or works out regularly what happens if they take a two-week break from their daily or alternate-day exercise routine – they will tell you it takes a few days again to get back to the same ease with which they were exercising before the break. The same applies to your meditation practice to some extent.

Another important point is to commit to your practice and stick to it, instead of trying different things every other day or trying to mix different techniques. At different times different masters may have given various techniques or instructions depending on who their students were, but don't get confused with that. See what is relevant for you and what works.

Sticking to one practice, at least for a considerable amount of time, will allow you to progress in the practice and reach somewhere. It will give you results. Trying something new or different every few days is like digging one metre in a thousand different places and wondering why you are not finding any water. Try digging one thousand metres in any place and you will definitely find water! So, sticking to a practice, being regular and honouring it can greatly help you to progress on your inward journey. And if you still feel that you don't have the time, you need to make time and see that this will benefit you so much more than almost all the other things that you are spending your time on. As long as you still have plenty of time to worry, get stressed, get upset or get depressed, you need to wake up and see that you definitely also have the time – and should take out the time – for a meditation practice.

If you feel in the beginning that your meditation is boring, just know that it is just a phase you are going through, because you are not yet really resting and you are still waiting for something to happen, you still want to engage the mind. Learning to meditate is a beautiful journey of learning to love being quiet and still for some time, of learning to love doing nothing, of learning to love this present moment, and to let the mind settle fully. It is a journey that will open up a whole new dimension of joy to you that is much more profound and long-lasting than what you have been used to till now.

Remember, meditation is a skill that comes by committed practice, not by 'knowing' something intellectually. So, unlike most mindfulness exercises, you don't have to focus, concentrate or visualize anything. All you need to do is stop doing – moving from effort to effortlessness. You are consciously giving your mind a break from all the worrying, thinking and planning that it is so used to doing, and you are allowing it to slow down and recharge.

Now that you are starting your meditation practice, it is also important to remember not to compare your experiences with that of other people, or with things you have heard or read somewhere. Because even though such experiences – seeing colours or a bright light, hearing sounds – may happen at some point, they are just that, experiences, and most of them are subjective. Trying to create such experiences, getting attached to them or taking them as a benchmark for your progress on the path of meditation will only confuse or distract you, or even worse, cause you to get frustrated, making you leave the practice altogether. Remember, meditation is not about the experiences, it is about the experiencer.

So then how do you know that you are making progress? What are indications that you are getting closer to your goal, and that your meditation practice is starting to bear fruits? When you feel fresher afterwards, and when you start noticing that in a subtle way that sense of joy, enthusiasm, peace and freedom starts increasing in your life.

Have you ever wondered what real peace is? What real peace of mind is? It is a mind that is naturally focused, in the sense that it is not scattered. It is a state where the mind is effortlessly focused on this very moment, on what is happening right now. When you are totally with what is happening right now that is real peace. It is when somewhere, subtly, you feel that this moment is not okay, that your mind goes off to the past or the future. Real peace is when you are here and now because it is okay.

In the same way, real freedom is freedom from the past and from the future, where you are comfortable in this moment. Because if this moment is not okay, if it is not perfect, there will always be some desire that comes up. After all, a desire means simply that: that the present moment, that what is here right now, is not how it should be. And any desire, whatever they may be, will not allow you to go deep in meditation and will hinder your quest for peace. You can keep sitting with your eyes closed, but your mind will keep going on its own trip and meditation will not happen. So, when we apply all the principles that we have learned in this book to transcend the desires during our meditation, you will find that this sense of acceptance, peace, freedom and joy starts to pervade other parts of your life as well, and more and more you will find that they become a part of you, even during your day-to-day activities.

Normally for as long as we are awake during the day, we keep looking outward. We engage ourselves in all kinds of activities, whether it is doing our work, talking, experiencing or thinking, and all this tires and drains us, however nice it may be. Except meditation. In meditation we take a break from all these activities of the body and mind, and we stop looking outward for a moment. When we start looking inward, it brings such rest, relaxation and relief, and that is exactly what the world needs today.

There is such tremendous uncertainty, fear, tension and depression in the world today, and sadly enough the global pandemic is just one of the many factors. Amidst all these challenges that the world is facing, and that we are facing on a personal level, we need a tool to stay afloat, something that will carry us through until we find solid ground again. Meditation can be this tool to survive, that allows us to dig deeper within ourselves and find our inner spiritual strength.

We are fortunate to be living in a time where the ancient wisdom that has been handed down to us in the tradition from thousands of years, and that had been authenticated by the scriptures and the experience of so many masters and practitioners over the ages, is inspiring researchers in leading institutions across the world to look at the benefits it brings to our lives with an open and scientific mind. The various benefits of meditation are too numerous to mention here, but now that even institutions like Harvard, Yale and many others have published well-researched papers on its manifold benefits, it should suffice to say that meditation as a practice has finally been welcomed as an ancient boon for our modern-day problems. For too long we have neglected the importance of knowing how to manage our mind, emotions, and the vital role these play in all aspects of our lives.

I remember the great tsunami that happened in 2004

the day after Christmas, that went down as one of the deadliest ones in recent history. Volunteers of The Art of Living and its sister organization the International Association for Human Values immediately rushed to the most heavily affected areas in India and Sri Lanka. Amongst them where some of my friends, and in the weeks and months that followed, they shared with me about the programs and initiatives we were doing there for the survivors of the tsunami, and one thing they mentioned really stuck with me.

They told me how people got the material aid they needed very quickly, as there were so many national and international humanitarian organizations that had rushed to their aid. But even though they got the food and medicines that they required, people weren't able to eat. They couldn't even sleep at night because they were so traumatized due to what had happened. This was an aspect that is often overlooked when providing aid, and it is where organizations like The Art of Living really make a difference.

Most of the survivors had lived on the seashore all their lives, and their whole life and livelihood revolved around and depended on the ocean. Most of them were fishermen or involved in some work related to the fishing trade. But now that the ocean, that had provided for them like a mother all their lives had suddenly turned into their greatest enemy, it was too much for them to digest. The one that had supported their lives till date, had suddenly taken away their homes, their boats and many of their near and dear ones. Many people had lost their father, mother, children or other relatives in that one moment of pure destruction. And it had left them so traumatized that they could not even sleep at night, as the sound of the waves and the ocean that had been their lullaby all their life, now carried with it nothing but the memory of the terror that the tsunami brought with it, and everything that it had successively taken away from them.

They had been provided with all the material aid and support they required, but it was almost pointless. People couldn't eat, couldn't sleep, and couldn't pick up their lives again. However, after several sessions of some of the breathing techniques and meditation people shared that they were able to sleep again at night. The sound of the waves and ocean was no longer traumatizing them – and after some more time they could actually go back into the sea again and pick up their lives as they knew best – as fishermen. They had been able to regain their inner strength and connect with the peace, stability and confidence that had been with them all along, and that nobody can take away. They were able to let go of the trauma, fear, despair and anger that had overpowered them completely.

They may have lost everything they had depended on for their security and stability till then, be it their family, their social support, their savings, their home, or their job, but the true strength and peace had remained untouched, as it lay safely deep within them. But in order to find it, access it and tap into it, they had to look inward. And so, do we.

Wisdom Sutras

- Wisdom is understanding why the practice is important and acting on it.
- For the practice to bear fruit, it needs to be done regularly with honour and commitment.

10-Minute Exercise

Take a strong commitment to start your meditation practice tomorrow itself. It is ideal to practice twice a day, once in the morning before breakfast, and once in the evening before dinner, but if that doesn't work out, don't make that an excuse to not do it. Anytime is a good time for meditation, except maybe right after a meal. Even if twice a day is initially difficult, make sure that you practice at least once a day, to get regular with your practice and to progress.

To have even better results from your practice, it would be good to fix a time for your meditation and try to stick to that time most of the days, if not all, especially to begin with. If that means you need to get up a little earlier so that you can squeeze it in before breakfast and heading out to the office, set your alarm and plan accordingly. If you are planning your meditation at any other time of the day, but you are having difficulty finding the time – or you feel that you don't have the time at all – then for the next one or two days keep noting down what you actually spend your time on. This is a very interesting exercise that can be a real eye-opener. You will find that the amount of time you spend just browsing the internet, Facebook, Instagram, Twitter, or YouTube, or any other social media, is actually much more than you had imagined. Add to this the time you spend watching movies, TV serials, as well as the time that you are just gossiping or complaining or worrying. Now take all that time, and decide to reduce it by 20-30 minutes, that you will instead invest in actually feeling better, happier, more rested and more peaceful, meaning, your meditation practice.

And may it be the beginning of a journey full of beauty, joy and peace, that never whither and that you carry with you wherever you go and share with whoever you meet.

Continuing the Journey: What Next?

Chances are that you can more or less place yourself in any of the following three categories of people who picked up this book and successfully completed reading it, and practising some, or all, of the exercises provided.

The first is someone who is new to meditation. You have started your practice, but you feel that you could use a little extra help to really get into it and settle the mind a little faster and more easily.

What would really benefit you, in this case, is to explore learning some of the pranayamas or breathwork techniques that I also have been practising for the last twenty years. It is a selection of a few very effective techniques that we teach in the Meditation and Breath Workshop of The Art of Living. The Sudarshan Kriya, which is a rhythmic breathing technique taught by Gurudev Sri Sri Ravi Shankar, has proven an invaluable tool for me in the last two decades of my meditation practice. We have certified trainers across the world who conduct these programs, and to locate upcoming workshops near you, you could just visit the global website of The Art of Living.

I also conduct these programs, and to find out more about my upcoming workshops, keep an eye on the event calendar on my website. Harnessing the power of the breath is one of the most effective ways to quieten and energize our mind, as I had already mentioned earlier in the book, and I can strongly recommend any practitioner of meditation to learn a few of these powerful breathwork techniques to complement and deepen their meditation practice and speed up their progress.

The second category of people that may have picked up this book are those that had already dabbled with mindfulness or meditation, but who never really got serious with their practice, or who were still looking for an effective and authentic meditation technique. This book would have given you a lot of practical knowledge and tools to get going, and you may have even been practising for a while now using what you have learned. However, you feel that you would like to go even deeper in your meditations by connecting with the practice and this ancient tradition on a more personal level. In this case I could strongly recommend joining one of the Sahaj Samadhi Meditation workshops that the Art of Living offers, as it provides practitioners with a personal mantra that is unique for you. These mantras have been handed down for ages in this ancient tradition, and the mantra given to you is a personalized tool that will help you to transcend the mind much more effortlessly and go even deeper in your meditation practice. It will also aid your progress on the spiritual path. I have personally practised this technique of meditation and have not come across any other meditation technique that is as effortless and effective. But, because you receive a unique mantra for your own practice, it needs to be received in the proper manner and given by a qualified teacher that is part of this ancient tradition. Those who are keen to learn more about this, or who would like to be initiated into this practice, can find more details on the Art of Living website. I regularly initiate practitioners into this ancient tradition of meditation, and more details of my programs can be found on my website as well.

The third category of people that you may find yourself in are those that have been practising meditation, whatever style or tradition you follow, and it is adding value to your life. However, you also feel that you would like to sometimes get away from all the daily hustle and bustle of your family or work environment and spend a few days to go much deeper and probe the subtler layers of your consciousness and being. At home, you may have the comfort and convenience of being able to create your own space, practice at your own convenient time and in whatever way you prefer, but at the same time it is still your home, with all its distractions and limitations.

This is the reason that in most traditions they also emphasized practising in a group, together, in a special location that is even more conducive to the practice. Because to deepen one's practice, to get into a structure and discipline, and to increase one's progress, practising in a group can be greatly beneficial. You will find most monasteries, ashrams, or meditation retreats set in an environment that is much more conducive than your busy home or office environment. And whenever your mind is wagging its tail, or your commitment is going down a little, you will find that being in a group will give you the support and occasional nudge in the back to keep going, and to pull through, especially on those days when you don't really feel like doing what you know you should be. This is the main reason why the Buddha also gave so much importance to the Sangha, or the community of practitioners, as it can be a support for one's practice.

It is to cater to this need as well, that we also conduct Advanced Meditation Programs under the Art of Living, which are special retreats, ranging from four to seven days, where in an environment conducive to meditation all your needs are taken care of. Light, nutritious meals and comfortable accommodation, coupled with no other distractions will allow you to fully focus on what you came for: to get away for a few days and go deep into your meditation practice. Experienced teachers like me will guide you through a range of profound and powerful guided meditations and other processes, as well as allow you to explore some of the ancient knowledge of the scriptures that will give you more understanding of the practices and the path. We have many advanced practitioners who make it a point to join such retreats two or three times a year, taking a few days from their busy schedules to refresh and rejuvenate themselves, and deepen their meditation practice.

Wherever you may find yourself, I wish you nothing but the best on your meditation journey, and I look forward to meeting you one day, and hear about your experiences! Let us not shy away from sharing this beautiful and much-needed knowledge with many more people, as these are trying times, and many are struggling to stay afloat.

For more about the programs of the global Art of Living Foundation, visit www.artofliving.org
For more information about my courses or to connect with me, visit www.swamipurnachaitanya.com